PATIENT VIOLENCE AND THE CLINICIAN

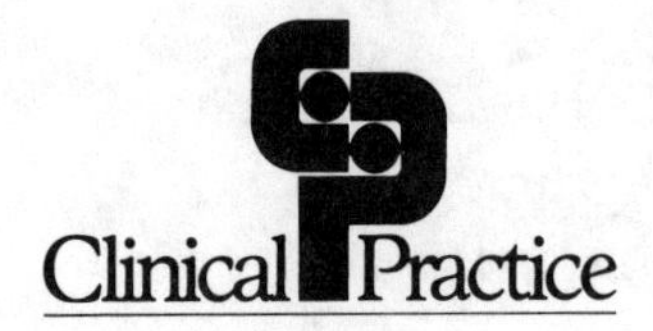

Number 30

Judith H. Gold, M.D., F.R.C.P.C.
Series Editor

PATIENT VIOLENCE AND THE CLINICIAN

Edited by

Burr S. Eichelman, M.D., Ph.D.

Anne C. Hartwig, J.D., Ph.D.

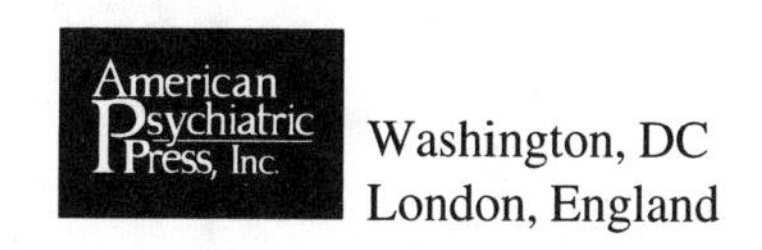

Washington, DC
London, England

Note: The authors have worked to ensure that all information in this book concerning drug dosages, schedules, and routes of administration is accurate as of the time of publication and consistent with standards set by the U.S. Food and Drug Administration and the general medical community. As medical research and practice advance, however, therapeutic standards may change. For this reason and because human and mechanical errors sometimes occur, we recommend that readers follow the advice of a physician who is directly involved in their care or the care of a member of their family.

Manufactured in the United States of America on acid-free paper
First Edition 98 97 96 95 4 3 2 1

American Psychiatric Press, Inc.
1400 K Street, N.W., Washington, DC 20005

Library of Congress Cataloging-in-Publication Data
Patient violence and the clinician / edited by Burr S. Eichelman and Anne C. Hartwig
p. cm. — (Clinical practice ; #30)
Includes bibliographical references and index.
ISBN 0-88048-454-3
1. Mental health personnel—Assaults against. 2. Violence in psychiatric hospitals. 3. Violence in hospitals. 4. Medical personnel—Assaults against. I. Eichelman, Burr S., 1943- II. Hartwig, Anne C. III. Series: Clinical practice ; no. 30
[DNLM: 1. Patients—psychology. 2. Mental Disorders—psychology. 3. Violence. 4. Physician-Patient Relations. W1 CL767J no. 30 1995 / WM 29.5 P298 1995]
RC439.4.P38 1995
362.1′1′0683—dc20
DNLM/DLC
for Library of Congress 94-36233
CIP

British Library Cataloguing in Publication Data
A CIP record is available from the British Library.

This book is dedicated to the memory of
Mary Ann Jerse, M.D., resident in psychiatry,
who was shot and killed in her outpatient
office by one of her patients.

Contents

Contributors

Kenneth L. Appelbaum, M.D.
Assistant Professor of Psychiatry, University of Massachusetts Medical School, Worcester, Massachusetts

Paul S. Appelbaum, M.D.
A. F. Zeleznik Professor of Psychiatry, University of Massachusetts Medical School, Worcester, Massachusetts

Renee L. Binder, M.D.
Professor in Residence, Department of Psychiatry, University of California, San Francisco, San Francisco, California

William R. Dubin, M.D.
Professor of Psychiatry, Temple University School of Medicine, and Associate General Director for Clinical Services, Belmont Hospital, Philadelphia, Pennsylvania

Burr S. Eichelman, M.D., Ph.D.
Professor and Chairman, Department of Psychiatry, Temple University School of Medicine, Philadelphia, Pennsylvania

David Fink, M.D.
Associate Director, Dissociative Disorders Unit, The Institute of Pennsylvania Hospital, Philadelphia, Pennsylvania

Paul Jay Fink, M.D.
Past President, American Psychiatric Association

Anne C. Hartwig, J.D., Ph.D.
Formerly Codirector, Institute of Law and Health Sciences, Temple School of Law, Department of Family Practice, Temple University School of Medicine, Philadelphia, Pennsylvania

David B. Langmeyer, Ph.D.
Consultant Psychologist, Raleigh, North Carolina, previously with the Department of Mental Health, State of North Carolina, Raleigh, North Carolina

Marilyn Lewis Lanza, R.N., D.N.Sc., Sc.
Associate Chief, Nursing Service for Research, Edith Nourse Rogers Memorial Veterans Hospital, Bedford, Massachusetts

John R. Lion, M.D.
Clinical Professor of Psychiatry, University of Maryland, Baltimore, Maryland

Gary J. Maier, M.D.
Clinical Associate Professor, University of Wisconsin, Madison, Wisconsin

Kenneth Tardiff, M.D., M.P.H.
Professor of Psychiatry and Public Health, Cornell Medical College, New York, New York

Gregory J. Van Rybroek, Ph.D., J.D.
Clinical Director, Mendota Mental Health Institute, Madison, Wisconsin

Introduction

to the Clinical Practice Series

Over the years of its existence the series of monographs entitled *Clinical Insights* gradually became focused on providing current, factual, and theoretical material of interest to the clinician working outside of a hospital setting. To reflect this orientation, the name of the Series has been changed to *Clinical Practice.*

The Clinical Practice Series will provide books that give the mental health clinician a practical, clinical approach to a variety of psychiatric problems. These books will provide up-to-date literature reviews and emphasize the most recent treatment methods. Thus, the publications in the Series will interest clinicians working both in psychiatry and in the other mental health professions.

Each year a number of books will be published dealing with all aspects of clinical practice. In addition, from time to time when appropriate, the publications may be revised and updated. Thus, the Series will provide quick access to relevant and important areas of psychiatric practice. Some books in the Series will be authored by a person considered to be an expert in that particular area; others will be edited by such an expert, who will also draw together other knowledgeable authors to produce a comprehensive overview of that topic.

Some of the books in the Clinical Practice Series will have their foundation in presentations at an annual meeting of the American Psychiatric Association. All will contain the most recently available information on the subjects discussed. Theoretical and scientific data will be applied to clinical situations, and case illustrations will be utilized in order to make the material even more relevant for the practitioner. Thus, the Clinical Practice Series should provide educational reading in a compact format especially designed for the mental health clinician–psychiatrist.

Judith H. Gold, M.D., F.R.C.P.C.
Series Editor
Clinical Practice Series

Clinical Practice Series Titles

Predictors of Treatment Response in Mood Disorders (#34)
Edited by Paul J. Goodnick, M.D.

Successful Psychiatric Practice in Changing Times: Current Dilemmas, Choices, and Solutions (#33)
Edited by Edward K. Silberman, M.D.

Alternatives to Hospitalization for Acute Psychiatric Treatment (#32)
Edited by Richard Warner, M.B., D.P.M.

Behavioral Complications in Alzheimer's Disease (#31)
Edited by Brian A. Lawlor, M.D.

Patient Violence and the Clinician (#30)
Edited by Burr S. Eichelman, M.D., Ph.D., and Anne C. Hartwig, J.D., Ph.D.

Effective Use of Group Therapy in Managed Care (#29)
Edited by K. Roy MacKenzie, M.D., F.R.C.P.C.

Rediscovering Childhood Trauma: Historical Casebook and Clinical Applications (#28)
Edited by Jean M. Goodwin, M.D., M.P.H.

Treatment of Adult Survivors of Incest (#27)
Edited by Patricia L. Paddison, M.D.

Madness and Loss of Motherhood: Sexuality, Reproduction, and Long-Term Mental Illness (#26)
Edited by Roberta J. Apfel, M.D., M.P.H., and Maryellen H. Handel, Ph.D.

Psychiatric Aspects of Symptom Management in Cancer Patients (#25)
Edited by William Breitbart, M.D., and Jimmie C. Holland, M.D.

Responding to Disaster: A Guide for Mental Health Professionals (#24)
Edited by Linda S. Austin, M.D.

Psychopharmacological Treatment Complications in the Elderly (#23)
Edited by Charles A. Shamoian, M.D., Ph.D.

Anxiety Disorders in Children and Adolescents (#22)
By Syed Arshad Husain, M.D., F.R.C.P.C., F.R.C.Psych., and
Javad Kashani, M.D.

Suicide and Clinical Practice (#21)
Edited by Douglas Jacobs, M.D.

Special Problems in Managing Eating Disorders (#20)
Edited by Joel Yager, M.D., Harry E. Gwirtsman, M.D., and Carole K. Edelstein, M.D.

Children and AIDS (#19)
Edited by Margaret L. Stuber, M.D.

Current Treatments of Obsessive-Compulsive Disorder (#18)
Edited by Michele Tortora Pato, M.D., and Joseph Zohar, M.D.

Benzodiazepines in Clinical Practice: Risks and Benefits (#17)
Edited by Peter P. Roy-Byrne, M.D., and Deborah S. Cowley, M.D.

Adolescent Psychotherapy (#16)
Edited by Marcia Slomowitz, M.D.

Family Approaches in Treatment of Eating Disorders (#15)
Edited by D. Blake Woodside, M.D., M.Sc., F.R.C.P.C., and Lorie Shekter-Wolfson, M.S.W., C.S.W.

Clinical Management of Gender Identity Disorders in Children and Adults (#14)
Edited by Ray Blanchard, Ph.D., and Betty W. Steiner, M.B., F.R.C.P.C.

New Perspectives on Narcissism (#13)
Edited by Eric M. Plakun, M.D.

The Psychosocial Impact of Job Loss (#12)
By Nick Kates, M.B.B.S., F.R.C.P.C., Barrie S. Greiff, M.D., and Duane Q. Hagen, M.D.

Office Treatment of Schizophrenia (#11)
Edited by Mary V. Seeman, M.D., F.R.C.P.C., and Stanley E. Greben, M.D., F.R.C.P.C.

Psychiatric Care of Migrants: A Clinical Guide (#10)
By Joseph Westermeyer, M.D., M.P.H., Ph.D.

Family Involvement in Treatment of the Frail Elderly (#9)
Edited by Marion Zucker Goldstein, M.D.

Measuring Mental Illness: Psychometric Assessment for Clinicians (#8)
Edited by Scott Wetzler, Ph.D.

Juvenile Homicide (#7)
Edited by Elissa P. Benedek, M.D., and Dewey G. Cornell, Ph.D.

The Neuroleptic Malignant Syndrome and Related Conditions (#6)
By Arthur Lazarus, M.D., Stephan C. Mann, M.D., and Stanley N. Caroff, M.D.

Anxiety: New Findings for the Clinician (#5)
Edited by Peter Roy-Byrne, M.D.

Anxiety and Depressive Disorders in the Medical Patient (#4)
By Leonard R. Derogatis, Ph.D., and Thomas N. Wise, M.D.

Family Violence: Emerging Issues of a National Crisis (#3)
Edited by Leah J. Dickstein, M.D., and Carol C. Nadelson, M.D.

Divorce as a Developmental Process (#2)
Edited by Judith H. Gold, M.D., F.R.C.P.C.

Treating Chronically Mentally Ill Women (#1)
Edited by Leona L. Bachrach, Ph.D., and Carol C. Nadelson, M.D.

Foreword

The violent patient inflicting injuries on psychiatrists and other mental health professionals has become a highly visible problem. Injuries to caretakers when the violent patient is brought to emergency rooms or admitted involuntarily to hospitals also occur. The problem of clinician safety was given a great deal of attention by the American Psychiatric Association when a task force was created to address this issue in 1988. Although we wish to be cautious about escalating negative stereotypes and stigma against the mentally ill, we also want to alert psychiatrists and other mental health professionals that patients could be dangerous and that there are techniques that can be used to protect oneself and to protect patients from harming themselves or others. We realize that, unfortunately, the media pay a disproportionate amount of attention to the relatively few violent acts carried out by violent patients. However, despite the media coverage, we believe that clinician safety is a significant issue that has been inadequately covered in the training of clinicians.

This very timely volume is an outgrowth of the work done by members of the task force who were appointed because of their recognized expertise in this area and the collaboration of experts outside of the task force. The editors have assembled a significant and important group of authors who open up the subject and provide essential clinical descriptions and excellent advice about how physicians, nurses, and other health care professionals should handle problems of weapons, physical abuse, and verbal abuse. The authors in this book further address the unique problems of female clinicians and patient assaults, particularly since there is a growing number of women entering psychiatry and these problems for female clinicians and safety have not been specifically or significantly addressed.

It is also enormously important that persons working in the field have some understanding of the magnitude of the problem and that we all recognize that this issue is pervasive—not because a large percentage of mentally ill patients are violent, but because the average physician sees a significant number of potentially violent patients either during his or her residency or in a lifetime of practice. It is of utmost practicality to know how to deal with potentially violent individuals. What will be revealed most cogently in this excellent book are the reactions of the treating therapist: the fear, the concern, the post-event feelings and reactions, the guilt, the sense of inadequacy, the review of the situation to find errors, in short, all of the nuances of ordinary therapeutic interaction. These nuances escalate when one of the parties (e.g., the patient) becomes a negative force, someone who no longer stimulates empathy but rather stimulates the therapist's anger, rage, and vindictiveness. How therapists feel and react in such times is described in the chapter on ethical issues. In addition, a controversial response, namely, prosecution as a response to violence by psychiatric patients, is discussed.

This is a comprehensive book on a timely problem. The authors represent a special group of experts who lead us through the dimensions of an issue that every psychiatrist, psychologist, social worker, and psychiatric nurse must face at some point in their professional lives.

Paul Jay Fink, M.D.
Past President
American Psychiatric Association

Acknowledgments

We thank T. Callaghan, E. Brown, and D. Tucker for their assistance in the typing of the manuscripts and the preparation of the text.

Chapter 1

A Commentary on Ethical Perspectives for Clinician Safety Application

Anne C. Hartwig, J.D., Ph.D.

The risk of violence by patients toward physicians is not a subject readily addressed either in research studies or in clinical training. Clinicians are left to devise for themselves protocol that will be sufficient to ensure their own personal safety and physical property while not encroaching on the special trust relationship between physician and patient. There are few published guidelines developed with the specific aim of meeting the needs of physicians. This is especially true for clinicians who have an increased risk of harm from potentially violent patients. There is virtually no well-known source for physicians to turn to when struggling with the problem of potential violence. The relatively few resources available do not comprehensively deal with the complex issue and leave the clinician to struggle on his or her own.

In the area of physician safety and patient fiduciary duties, a discussion of ethical principles is invaluable. It is, indeed, in the *patients' and physicians'* interests to discuss thoroughly, if not comprehend, the contribution that ethics, as a means of facilitating decision making, can make. Regardless of which principles govern the decision, ethical algorithms offer physicians a "safe" process in which to articulate their fears and concerns and, more importantly, balance their needs in response to the patient's mental and emotional crises. It is unfortunate that a discussion of ethical principles is often treated as a separate topic, outside of and usually devoid of practical, real-world application. An understanding of an applied ethics and of its contribution to decision making has been for the most part relegated to one or two "token" chapters or paragraphs.

Therefore, the purpose of this brief introductory chapter is to suggest that the relationship among acts, values, and faith may provide a basis for a decision-making model as illustrated in Figure 1–1. This chapter also presents perspectives of both deontological and teleological models in an attempt to challenge the reader to refer back to the perspectives as the reader moves through the remainder of the book. It is not intended that the reader be fully conversant with ethical dialogue at the conclusion of the book. However, it is intended that the reader use the perspectives presented as a means of dealing with decision making in the area of promoting physician safety while respecting the physician-patient relationship.

Ethics in Clinical Decision Making

It is the thesis of this chapter that ethics in clinical decision making is a process based on a logical framework as exemplified in Figure 1–2. It is a process that begins with an understanding of a clinical situation and an understanding of ethical principles that apply to that situation. Ethical decision making is rarely the adoption of an ethical principle versus not adopting a principle. It is usually a dilemma in decision making caused by the conflict between two or more competing ethical principles. The actual ethical *process* is a weighing of these principles

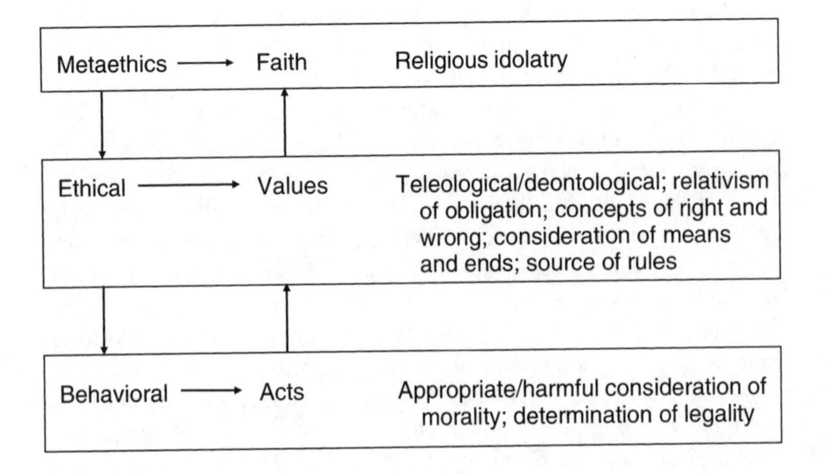

Figure 1–1. Suggested relationship among acts, values, and faith.

and an examination of how they may conflict with one another and even with the law. This weighing may be done individually, by the clinician alone. It may be done among colleagues, as in a practice group or with an inpatient staff. It may be done in a more formal setting, as within a hospital's ethics committee or human rights committee. Always, it is done within and reflective of the moral climate of the culture specific to the times.

It is this process, this dialogue, that cultivates an ethical environment. "Ethical" decisions may change over time through a differential weighing of particular principles. Ethical decision making is not a static process. This may be the most challenging corollary to this chapter's thesis.

Legal Versus Ethical Mandates

The boundary between legal mandate—what does the law dictate—and ethical principle is frequently so blurred as to be impossible to discern. Only if one accepts an absolute ethical posture "*always* to adhere to the law" as one might choose "*always* to tell the truth" can one equate legal action with ethical action. The implementation of various ethical principles, such as Kant's (1983) respect for persons or Mill's (1863) utilitarianism, under certain conditions might well run contrary to the law. Conversely, failure to act ethically may not break the law but may be ethically flawed behavior.

Legal mandates are often inappropriately exalted, by those who either fear the law or do not comprehend it, to lofty a place; liability

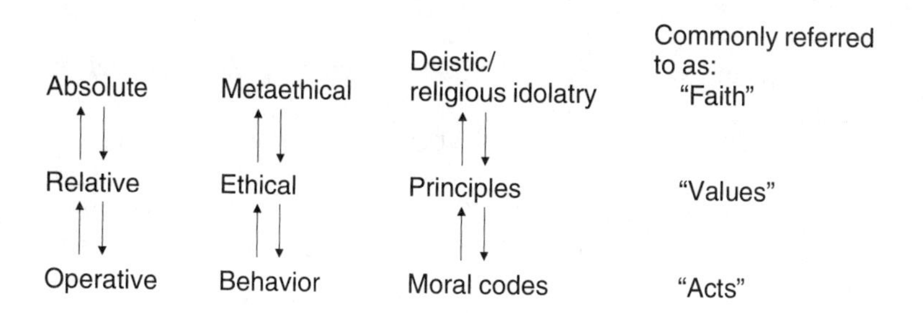

Figure 1–2. Logical framework.

often becomes the determinant of a decision. Similarly, legal feasibility may play too prominent a role in a discussion about what to do when conflicts involving rights and responsibilities arise. Legal feasibility is but one criterion for policy choice. As Dworkin (1986) argued, there is, inevitably, a moral dimension to an action at law. However, the law is an often slowly reactive institution, responding gradually to demands for change and obligated to answer to its constituents. In contrast, ethics as a process is available to all individuals, offering structure and principles that can be universally understood. Throughout this book, the process is invoked and embraced by clinicians as they develop protocols that will enable them to feel safe as they treat their patients.

Tools for the Ethical Process

Most of the ethical principles that must be weighed in the policy- and decision-making issues regarding clinician safety can be described as either teleological or deontological principles (Table 1–1). These two categories of ethical principles often conflict when ethical behavior is attempted. Teleological, from the Greek root *telos* (end), principles look at the outcome. In contrast, deontological, from the Greek root

Table 1–1. System of values based on principles of ethical systems

Teleological	Deontological
Assessing human behavior in terms of its accomplishment, with a view toward desired ends or goals	Assessing human behavior in terms of the principles or responsibilities of the actor or agent
Utilitarian theories	Kantian duties
There is intrinsic good	Do good from duty and not inclination
Intrinsic good can be measured	An action based on duty has worth because of the maxim on which it rests
If measured, good is maximizable	Good is achievable only through duty
End may be predicted and calculated	The categorical imperative is without calculus
Egalitarian effort is related to ends	Duty should be universal

deon (that which is obligatory), principles, focus on the nature of the behavior, not on its outcome.

Teleological Perspectives

These ethical positions are often described in the context of "distributive justice," or the ethical distribution of resources. Although such distribution is often considered in relation to an allocation of physical resources ranging from wealth to the use of hospital beds, it can also be envisioned in relation to clinician attention or time or even policy focus.

Utilitarianism

The most commonly used philosophical construct in medicine is utilitarianism. John Stuart Mill (1957) suggested a utilitarian model that proposes an ethical construct that is often used in decisions that provide the greatest good for the greatest number. This use of Mill's model is readily apparent in medicine in the area of allocation of resources. Arguably, the health care system in the United States reflects this dimension of utilitarianism. However, the needs of the individual patient may fall outside the calculus; the individual concerns of the physician may, similarly, be set aside in a system so heavily imbued with the balancing of great over small and significant over insignificant numbers.

A second dimension of utilitarianism exhorts a view to the end results over the means employed. This "end justifies the means" shortcut is also used in medicine, usually as a rationale for requiring the public to comply with specific health preventive measures as in the example of mandatory vaccinations against infectious diseases, an infringement on personal liberty for the benefit of society. Mill's (1957) utilitarian principle is a *group* or societal principle. In this regard, it is not easily applied to *individual* problems and solutions. Sometimes the value of individual intervention is measured by "the best interests of the patient" standard. This standard is not a utilitarian ethical principle. It is a statement of purpose and justification but should not be confused with utilitarian-teleological maxims. Its ethical derivation can be derived from Kantian deontological premises discussed later.

Rawlsian Ethics

John Rawls (1971) proposed an ethical allocation process that would "distribute" resources to the most disadvantaged and disenfranchised persons in society. The distributive justice advocated by Rawls is also frequently seen in medicine in mental health in the establishment of free clinics, mental health crisis lines, and other examples guaranteeing access to services. As with Mill, it is difficult to apply Rawls' thinking to an individual patient who has access to care but who may jeopardize his or her treatment because of potential violent acts.

At first glance, it appears virtually impossible to think of Rawlsian justice in the context of physician safety. Consider, however, that if the ultimate achievement, from an ethical perspective, is individual liberty—as a resource—for all patients, then *any* decision or intervention that ultimately results in the recognition of individual autonomy is indeed defensible, according to principles of Rawlsian distributive justice. To be judged or viewed as competent, in charge of one's life, is then the ultimate goal of therapy. All interventions that move an individual toward that goal are consonant with utilitarianism. This appears to be a sound rationale from a patient advocate point of view. Concrete corollaries of this principle would include the physician referring the patient to another clinician because of safety concerns or, at the extreme, even deciding to bring legal action against the patient because of the patient's violent acts toward the physician. In both the act of referral and of legal action, the physician may be deemed to be acting within the constructs of furthering the patient's individual autonomy balanced with responsibility—a solid ethical goal.

Marxism. Marxism's distribution of resources, from each according to ability to each according to need (Marx 1938), appears readily applicable to the physician safety problem. This ethical perspective exhorts physicians to look at the needs of the patients, a position that is necessary in decisions about what to do in a specific situation. Not only does this become an economic issue of distributing financial resources to violent, mentally ill persons beyond their own ability to generate these resources, but it also suggests an obligatory sharing of other resources, including behavioral resources or coping strategies (e.g., to reduce violence), by others, such as the therapist with his or her patient.

Deontological Perspectives

The foremost philosophical construct within deontology is the principle of respect for persons as detailed by Kant (1983). In contrast to utilitarian ethics, Kant maintained that one should "act so as to treat humanity in oneself and others only as an end in itself, and never merely as a means" (Wick 1983). For Kant, an act is not moral unless duty is behind it. The principle embodies the idea of persons as rational beings worthy of respectful treatment. It assumes the rationality or potential for rationality for all and precludes the possibility of treating the person as an object (Kant 1983). The embedded principle, respect for persons, is the duty owed to all persons. A physician, acting as the agent, acts out of *duty* without regard to the potential benefits that may be received. Thus, the moral worth of an action does not depend on its consequences but on the ethical value of the principle (Kant 1983).

Kant and the deontological constructs of respect for persons and duty do not necessarily mean, however, that one should put oneself in danger. In fact, deontology and Kant, in particular, maintain that there is a duty to secure one's own happiness and to preserve one's own life. Arguably, actions taken by a clinician to preserve his or her own life are consonant with the deontological perspective.

Pragmatically, having "good intentions" alone is not sufficient for moral behavior. Monastic—unifocal—systems, such as Kant's (1983) ethical formalism, and utilitarianism must be combined or contrasted in deliberations about what is or is not an ethical course of action, what action was intended by the principal actors in an event, and what results ensued. It is not enough to add ethical considerations to the frill of the decision-making process itself. Ethical behavior involves weighing all the considerations morally relevant to every alternative course of action (Taylor 1975). Indeed, disregarding ethical reasoning in taking a clinical action may lead to untoward consequences.

For the clinician, a deontological principle is *primum non nocere* (first do no harm). Even the role of the hospital or clinician acting as parens patriae can be considered as a deontological duty to ensure the welfare of patients entrusted to care. This might require ensuring health and safety even (particularly) in situations where it is most difficult to do so.

Deontological principles can conflict just as deontological and teleological principles can conflict. The tension between respecting a patient's confidentiality—a corollary of Kant's respect for persons—comes directly into conflict with primum non nocere when the patient names an intended victim for future proximate violence. Both maintaining confidentiality and providing a Tarasoff warning to the potential victim are traceable to solid ethical principles. What is stressed in this chapter, however, is that truly ethical clinical care and decision making attempt to integrate or balance ethical principles for a given clinical situation. It is this process of weighing, balancing, and deliberating with colleagues and society that is at the very heart of ethical care.

An Application of Ethical Principles

Once some background regarding ethical principles has been established, one can proceed to an examination of the complexity of weighing and balancing such principles for a particular case to generate an ethically driven clinical decision. The two cases described here highlight the ethical complexity of what could otherwise be regarded as reflexive (i.e., knee-jerk) clinical decisions.

> *Case A.* A patient who has been in therapy for a substantial period of time with Dr. Y. has made indirect threats to the therapist in the last several therapy sessions. During this session, he becomes enraged. He picks up an ashtray and hurls it at Dr. Y., breaking a window. He storms out of the office. Dr. Y. is concerned about his own safety and believes that the patient remains potentially violent.

1. Is the physician ethically bound to reveal to others the patient's verbal threats? Arguably, using Mill's (1957) logic, the only time that intervention is, in fact, justified is when a danger to others exists. However, using one deontological maxim, the physician has a duty to do no harm to the patient.
2. If the therapist reveals the patient's threats to the authorities and the patient is subsequently arrested, arguably "harm" has been done. How far does the maxim go? Does the therapist need to weigh or balance the apparently competing interests? Kant might argue that if there are moral imperatives and do no harm is a moral imperative, then no balancing is required. The problem is that there is also a maxim to preserve one's own safety. Which maxim is takes precedence?

3. How does one integrate legal responsibility as regards confidentiality, commitment statutes, and Tarasoff legislation with moral duty? Just what are the limits for preserving confidentiality? How and when is a breach of confidentiality justified?
4. What ethical duties are owed by the clinician to colleagues and support staff who might be involved with this client?
5. Does the clinician "owe" a duty to his or her own family that impinges on his or her clinical intervention at this time?
6. What if the patient has alluded to violence against the clinician's family? The clinician is forced to balance the ethical corollaries of the fiduciary relationship with his or her patient with the quite different duties that stem from a family relationship.
7. Does the clinician have different obligations to colleagues than to his or her own family?

Case B. A second-year psychiatric resident has been treating a noncompliant schizophrenic male patient. There is no protocol or clinical policy concerning violent patients; in fact, there are no written procedures that address safety precautions. The senior supervising staff has discussed such a protocol but has been unable to come to any resolution about specific issues.

After a hiatus of several months, the patient requests an unscheduled visit in the early morning hours before the clinic is formally open. The resident does not inform anyone of the patient's request. The patient arrives at the clinic, and the resident takes him back to her office. He shoots and kills her and then kills himself.

1. What are the duties owed by the senior staff to the residents and trainees? Are there legal principles involved (e.g., fiduciary duties)? Are these duties also ethical (e.g., respect for persons)? Did the attending staff have a duty, greater than exercised, to review such cases with the resident? Should enhanced training have occurred within such a program? If both were true, what other training modules or supervisory topics should have been deleted?
2. Did the resident have some responsibility to the patient in seeing him at an unusual hour? Is this responsibility reduced for the noncompliant patient? Is there any ethical duty to treat noncompliant patients? Yet, tolerating degrees of noncompliance is a means of respecting the autonomy of another person. Does this

endangerment differ in relation to a compliant versus a noncompliant patient?

Kantian principles may bring the duty questions into sharper focus by examining the nature of respect for persons and the assumptions that all of us must make as to just what behaviors constitute affording an individual "respect."

These cases contain far more questions and issues than those briefly highlighted earlier. Further, as one proceeds through the subsequent chapters, many additional ethical dilemmas should become evident.

In considering "high-risk" patient populations, should such populations receive greater mental health resources than less violent groups? Should they receive less "respect" as regards privacy and confidentiality or even the clinician's willingness to implement some degree of risk taking in the therapy?

Should certain clinicians (e.g., those frequently assaulted) receive greater resources in staffing or training, or should they be restricted in their clinical autonomy and more closely monitored? Should trainees in the early phases of their training no longer be assigned the most dangerous patients? What if the assignment is made within closely supervised settings? Is there an ethical duty for experienced clinicians to assume the direct care of the most dangerous patients?

As in cases A and B, what are the ethical boundaries and rationale for breaking confidentiality when verbal threats or weapons are involved? How does one justify restricting liberty through a ward "lockup" to process staff feelings and meet clinician needs while transiently suppressing the need for freedom and autonomy of the patient?

In the ethical distribution of resources, would Rawlsian theory justify hospital funding for an employee assistance program to address the needs of assaulted staff at the expense of limiting the budget for nursing positions on a violent unit? How about taking staff from a nonviolent "chronic unit"? How does a hospital management weigh the expenditure for the establishment of a ward alarm system against the remodeling of a quiet but dilapidated geriatric psychiatry unit?

In prosecuting a violent patient, is the ethical motive behind this action to encourage the patient to acknowledge his or her responsibility for nonviolence or is it to gain some retribution for staff, treating the patient as an object? The ethical stance for prosecution might be justified by Kant in the former position, but not in the latter position, even though the action is the same.

The process of ethical review surrounding the topics within this book will certainly generate varying points of view. It may also serve to raise consciousness about duty and responsibility. Such concepts are often misunderstood by individuals who feel pressured to "do the right thing." Further, a lively discussion about ethics may enhance a process of decision making that incorporates legal responses, placing these in a more reasonable mode and allowing them to be viewed in a more reasonable light. Finally, ethical perspectives are a sound basis on which to formulate policy. In fostering ethical debate, clinicians have an opportunity to rehearse their responses and devise reflective action grounded in ethical principles.

References

Dworkin R: Law's Empire. Cambridge, MA, Harvard University Press, 1986

Kant I: The Metaphysics of Morals. Translated by Ellington JW. Indianapolis, IN, Hackett, 1983

Marx K: Critique of the Gotha Program. New York, International Publishing, 1938

Mill JS: Utilitarianism (1863). Indianapolis, IN, Bobbs-Merrill, 1957

Rawls J: A Theory of Justice. Cambridge, MA, Harvard University Press, 1971

Taylor PW: Principles of Ethics: An Introduction. Belmont, CA, Wadsworth Press, 1975

Wick WA: Introduction: Kant's moral philosophy, in Immanuel Kant: Ethical Philosophy. Indianapolis, IN, Hackett, 1983

Chapter 2

The Risk of Being Attacked by Patients: Who, How Often, and Where?

Kenneth Tardiff, M.D., M.P.H.

In this chapter, I review the literature on patient attacks toward clinicians. My intent is to alert clinicians about the danger and risk of patient attacks and to discuss potential safety measures for clinicians who evaluate and treat violent patients.

Studies have found that approximately 40% of psychiatrists report having been physically attacked by patients one or more times. There were several studies in the early 1970s. For example, Whitman and colleagues (1976) sent a questionnaire to 184 mental health workers in psychiatry, psychology, and social work in Cincinnati, Ohio, asking about the number of patients seen in the 1972 calendar year, the number the therapist felt posed threats to the therapist, and the number who actually were assaultive toward the therapist. Of the 101 respondents, 80 worked primarily in outpatient settings and 21 in inpatient settings. Of the total group of respondents, 79% reported at least one incident in which a patient posed a threat to others, and 43% of the respondents reported at least one incident in which the clinician felt personally threatened. When asked whether they had been physically attacked during that year, 24% of the respondents replied that they had been attacked. Psychiatrists appeared at higher risk than other clinicians, with 34% reporting having been attacked compared with 7% of the psychologists and 20% of the social workers. There were 3,810 patients seen by the psychiatrists during the year. Of these, 416 patients (11%) were perceived by the psychiatrists as posing some assaultive threat to other persons. Of the total patients seen, 91 (2.4%) posed a direct threat to the psychiatrist, and 33 (.87%) assaulted the psychiatrists. Thus, Whitman and colleagues concluded that although the percentage of patients assaulting psychiatrists was low, the risk increased as therapists saw more patients.

Tardiff and Maurice (1977) surveyed 210 psychiatrists who worked in Vancouver, Canada. The response rate was 48% with 100 usable responses. Most of the psychiatrists were involved in direct patient care in outpatient settings, and 13% were in residency training. Of these psychiatrists, 40% reported one or more personal attacks during their careers.

In 1975, Madden and colleagues (1976) sent questionnaires to 115 psychiatrists around the Baltimore, Maryland, area who held full-time or part-time positions at the University of Maryland, including those in private practice, medical school positions, and state hospital, forensic, and prison positions. There was a 100% response rate; 42% reported being attacked one or more times during his or her career. Most were attacked by patients in treatment and continued to see these patients after the attack occurred. In the late 1970s, Ruben and colleagues (1980) interviewed 31 second- and third-year psychiatry residents in Los Angeles, California. Fifteen residents (48%) reported being attacked at least once during their years in the residency program.

In the beginning of the 1980s, Hatti and colleagues (1982) mailed a questionnaire to 650 psychiatrists in Philadelphia, Pennsylvania, listed in a directory of physicians. In addition, the questionnaire was sent to 75 psychiatrists in London, England. In Philadelphia, 312 psychiatrists responded; 20% said they had been physically attacked by patients one or more times. In London, 45 psychiatrists responded; 24% said they had been attacked by patients. Bernstein (1981) surveyed mental health professionals in San Diego, California, including 171 psychiatrists, 252 psychologists, 244 social workers, and 404 counselors in marital, family, and child therapy. The overall response rate was 46%. The psychiatrists reported that 52% had been attacked by patients and 61% had been threatened. The other professionals reported lower rates—10% having been attacked and 32% having been threatened by patients. The respondents, in even greater proportions, expressed a fear of being attacked.

In a survey of professionals in outpatient treatment settings, Reid and Kang (1986) mailed a questionnaire to 470 psychiatrists, 150 psychologists, and 350 family practice physicians. Of the psychiatrists and family practitioners, 33% responded; 66% of the psychologists responded. Reid and Kang limited their study of attacks to those they defined as serious (i.e., resulting in 1 or more days missed from work). They found that 3% of the psychiatrists and family practitioners and 1% of the psychologists reported having been attacked during their careers using this definition of serious attacks.

A survey of psychiatrists in outpatient settings was conducted by Dubin and colleagues (1988), who sent questionnaires to psychiatrists in Pennsylvania, New Jersey, and Delaware. Of the respondents, 91 reported having been attacked in an outpatient setting.

In contrast, studies of mental health professionals predominantly within inpatient settings show that the proportion of nurses and other staff attacked by patients is greater than that of psychiatrists, psychologists, and social workers. In 1986, Carmel and Hunter (1989) reviewed injuries to staff in a large forensic hospital in California and focused on injuries that resulted in lost workdays, loss of consciousness, restriction of work or motion, termination of employment, transfer to another job, or receiving medical treatment other than first aid. Of 749 ward nursing staff, including registered nurses, supervisors, and psychiatric technicians, 6% reported attacks directed toward them by patients, and 10% reported injuries sustained while attempting to control patients. Of 106 psychiatric technician trainees, 2% reported direct attacks, and 4% reported injuries while attempting to control patients. The respondent psychiatrists, psychologists, social workers, and rehabilitation therapists reported no direct attacks, although 2% reported injuries sustained while controlling patients.

Lanza (1985) surveyed 99 nurses in a Veterans Administration hospital and found that 79% reported having been attacked by patients. Of the surveyed nurses, 21% reported never being attacked, 58% reported being attacked 1–3 times, 13% reported 4–6 incidents, 3% reported 7–10 times, and 4% reported being attacked by patients more than 10 times in their careers.

Reports from professionals in the National Health Service in England parallel the statistics in the United States (Mackay 1987). There were approximately 3,000 responses from professionals in various treatment settings. Of the respondents, 18% had been threatened by patients with a weapon, 11% had received injuries that required first aid, and 0.5% suffered injuries that required significant medical treatment. Of these injuries, 30% involved a weapon, and 10% of the victims were admitted to a hospital for treatment. Professionals working in psychiatric facilities were more likely than professionals in other health facilities to suffer injuries by patients. Of professionals in psychiatric settings, 31% had been threatened by patients, 12% had been threatened by a patient with a weapon, 27% had received injuries that required first aid, and 2% suffered injuries that required major medical treatment within 1 year. Considering professionals in all types of settings, physicians reported 19% threats, 3% weapons, 6% injuries requiring first aid, and 0.5% for major injuries.

The "target" of attacks by patients is related to the treatment setting. Psychiatrists are more likely to be attacked than psychologists, social workers, and other therapists in predominantly outpatient settings, although nurses are more likely to be targets of attack in inpatient settings. Another factor related to who is more likely to be attacked by patients is the youth and/or inexperience of clinicians. This is particularly true for psychiatric residents who have high rates of being attacked considering their short time being at risk. Most of the studies found no significant difference between male and female clinicians in terms of being victims of attacks. Madden and colleagues (1976) found that most of the attacks on clinicians were made during the early phases of their training by patients who were in active treatment. In a forensic state hospital, nursing and other staff recently hired were more often victims of direct attacks by patients than were more experienced staff (Carmel and Hunter 1989). Whether the increased number of attacks against new clinicians is related to a greater likelihood of their exposure to violent patients or the result of inexperience and lack of training is unclear. Tardiff (1974) found that younger psychiatrists are more likely to have contact with violent patients, presumably because they are on the front lines in emergency rooms and inpatient units. It may also be that they are more likely to accept difficult patients as they build their practices. Whitman and colleagues (1976) concluded that the more patients the therapist sees, the more threats and attacks he or she can expect.

Other researchers have found that the inexperience of clinicians does contribute to their being attacked by patients. Madden and colleagues (1976) found that more than half of the psychiatrists attacked by patients said they could have anticipated the attack. They said they acted in a provocative manner by making comments or interpretations that were unfavorably received by the patient, by refusing to meet a patient's request, and by setting either too many or not enough limits. Others felt they were too insistent that the patient confront upsetting

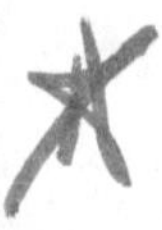

material or that transference and countertransference were not properly addressed in treatment. Hatti and colleagues (1982) confirmed the importance of dealing with interpersonal issues in decreasing the risk of being attacked by patients. Ruben and colleagues (1980) focused on residents who had been attacked and found that almost every resident felt that they frustrated the patient while setting limits (e.g., in admitting or not admitting a patient to the hospital or forcing medications). These authors suggested that this may have been due to a lack of knowledge as to how to set limits while minimizing frustration, but they also found that the personality of the resident, as in being irritable and outspoken, may have contributed to incidents of violence by patients.

A more direct measurement of the role of training in decreasing the likelihood of being attacked was done by Infantino and Musingo (1985), who studied the effect of a 3-day course for staff in a state hospital. The staff were taught to "defuse" potentially violent behavior verbally and, if necessary, to take nonoffensive physical action to control attacks. Of those trained, only one staff member (3%) was attacked during the study period, whereas 24 (37%) of those not trained were attacked.

Which patients are more likely to attack their therapists? As with violence in general, perpetrators are more likely to be male and in the younger age groups, at least under 30–40 years old (Hatti et al. 1982; Madden et al. 1976; Ruben et al. 1980). However, there were women and older patients who attacked clinicians. The most frequent diagnosis found among patients attacking clinicians was schizophrenia. Madden and colleagues found that 63.9% of those who attacked were schizophrenic patients and another 9% had other psychotic disorders. The remainder of those who attacked had personality disorders or fell into other diagnostic groups. Hatti and colleagues found that 52% of those who attacked were schizophrenic patients and that the most frequent chief complaints by patients were paranoid ideation and depression. Again, patients with personality disorders constituted a large proportion of the rest, namely 30%. Ruben and colleagues found that more than half of the patients who attacked were psychotic, but these authors did not specify the diagnosis. Two published case histories of attacks on psychiatrists in hospitals (one fatal and the other near-fatal) describe severe delusional problems in the schizophrenic patients who made the attacks (Annis and Baker 1986; La Brash and Cain 1984).

Dubin and colleagues (1988) found that 40% of the patients who attacked were schizophrenic, especially in the paranoid subgroup; 35% had personality disorders as primary diagnoses; and 10% were manic. There was no statistically significant difference between diagnosis and the seriousness of the attacks. The authors also gathered information about the characteristics of the therapy the patients were receiving; 36% of the patients had been in therapy for more than a year.

One final question concerns where clinicians are attacked. A simple answer is in all types of settings: inpatient units, outpatient offices, and even homes. Hatti and colleagues (1982) found half of the attacks on psychiatrists in practice took place in outpatient settings. When weapons were used, the attacks occurred in outpatient settings. Ruben and colleagues (1980) found a similar variety in the settings where psychiatric residents were attacked. Locations included outpatient departments, ward halls, doctors' offices, and physical examination rooms during examinations. Attacks usually involved available objects such as ashtrays, telephones, and books, or fists. Dubin and colleagues (1988) focused on attacks in outpatient settings and found that they occurred outside institutional settings (e.g., a community mental health center). For example, 36% (9 of 16 assaults with guns) occurred in office buildings and 13% in the psychiatrists' home offices. Only 23% of the psychiatrists attacked reported having taken any prior security precautions; of those, one-third failed to use the precautions during the attack.

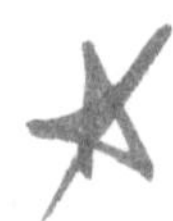

The responses of the clinicians who were attacked yield information that may minimize injury in the future. Whitman and colleagues (1976) categorized responses into 1) biological, as in the use of physical or chemical controls; 2) psychological, as in verbal responses or controls; and 3) social, as in the use of peer, institutional, or family influence. They observed that the clinicians tended to use only the response related to the way they generally treat patients. The authors suggested that there should be further training of clinicians aimed at a broader repertoire of responses to fit different situations. Hatti and colleagues (1982) found that physical force by staff was used to control the patients in 40% of the threatening episodes; 35% of psychiatrists talked with the patients until the violent confrontation remitted.

There have been few studies on the psychological impact of being threatened or physically injured. Lanza (1985) reported that 71% of nurses attacked by patients reported fairly severe to very severe emotional reactions to the assault. Approximately 45% said they did not expect to receive any support from their peers or the institution. Most of the nurses said they would expect that a victim would want to talk to someone about the assault, but 37% said it might be "unprofessional" to express one's feelings about the assault. Further conflict revealed a high degree of discomfort in caring for a patient who assaulted them. All of this points out the need for administration to have in place a program in which a victim can receive immediate peer support and the opportunity for longer term professional care to cope with the sequelae of violence.

In summary, attacks on clinicians by patients constitute a significant problem. Clinicians at greatest risk, regardless of discipline, are the young and the inexperienced. Training programs for clinicians to prevent or manage violence are usually aimed at staff on inpatient units and have demonstrated effectiveness. There is a need for formal, comprehensive education of psychiatric residents, other trainees, and practitioners in the mental health professions about safety and coping with threats and violence by patients. All clinicians regardless of place and type of practice should think about safety since attacks occur in a wide variety of outpatient as well as inpatient settings. It is the responsibility of the individual clinician and the institution to develop plans to enhance security and the safety of treatment settings. Last, attention should be given to the support and treatment of colleagues who are victims of violence by patients to address the personal and professional sequelae of violence.

References

Annis LV, Baker CA: A psychiatrist's murder in a mental hospital. Hosp Community Psychiatry 37:505–506, 1986

Bernstein HA: Survey of threats and assaults directed toward psychotherapists. Am J Psychother 35:542–549, 1981

Carmel H, Hunter H: Staff injuries from inpatient violence. Hosp Community Psychiatry 40:41–46, 1989

Dubin WR, Wilson SJ, Mercer C: Assaults against psychiatrists in outpatient settings. J Clin Psychiatry 49:338–345, 1988

Hatti S, Dubin WR, Weiss KJ: A study of circumstances surrounding patient assaults on psychiatrists. Hosp Community Psychiatry 33:660–661, 1982

Infantino JA, Musingo S: Assaults and injuries among staff with and without training in aggression control techniques. Hosp Community Psychiatry 36:1312–1314, 1985

La Brash L, Cain J: A near-fatal assault on a psychiatric unit. Hosp Community Psychiatry 35:168–169, 1984

Lanza ML: How nurses react to assault. J Psychosoc Nurs Ment Health Serv 23:6–11, 1985

Mackay CJ: Violence to Staff in the Health Services. London, Health and Safety Commission, National Health Service, 1987

Madden DJ, Lion JR, Penna MW: Assaults on psychiatrists by patients. Am J Psychiatry 133:422–425, 1976

Reid WH, Kang JS: Serious assaults by outpatients or former patients. Am J Psychother 40:594–600, 1986

Ruben I, Wolkon G, Yamamoto J: Physical attacks on psychiatric residents by patients. J Nerv Ment Dis 168:243–245, 1980

Tardiff K: A survey of psychiatrists in Boston and their work with violent patients. Am J Psychiatry 131:1008–1011, 1974

Tardiff K, Maurice WL: The care of violent patients by psychiatrists: a tale of two cities. Canadian Psychiatric Association Journal 22:83–86, 1977

Whitman RM, Armao BB, Dent OB: Assault on the therapist. Am J Psychiatry 133:426–431, 1976

Chapter 3

Women Clinicians and Patient Assaults

Renee L. Binder, M.D.

Although both women and men clinicians are assaulted, there are some gender differences, including pregnancy, that may affect a clinician's likelihood of being assaulted. In this chapter, I specifically focus on special issues related to women clinicians and patient assaults.

Incidence

Studies have shown that between 40% and 50% of psychiatrists will be assaulted by a patient during the course of their professional lives (Madden et al. 1976; Tardiff and Maurice 1977). Although there are no large-scale studies about the incidence of assaults against women clinicians, most of the studies that have been done suggest that women are, at least, at an equally high risk as men for being assaulted. In fact, there is only one study that suggests that women are at lower risk than men for being assaulted. In this study of women nursing staff, Levy and Harticollis (1976) reported that there were no incidents of violence on a unit staffed only by women. The authors hypothesized that violence-prone patients may find female nurses and aides less provocative than male staff and that women are more apt to rely on a nonaggressive manner and "feminine intuition" when confronted with threatening patients. Other studies have found women to be at an equal risk of being

---

Portions of this chapter were previously published in the *Bulletin of the Academy of Psychiatry and Law* 19:291–296, 1991. Used with permission.

assaulted as men. For example, in their study of psychiatric residents, Fink and colleagues (1991) showed that 41% of the residents had been assaulted, with no difference in the rates of assaults against men and women. Similarly, Whitman and colleagues (1976) surveyed psychotherapists (psychiatrists, psychologists, and social workers) and found no differences in threats or assaults against men and women. Moreover, in a forensic hospital setting, Carmel and Hunter (1989) found that the difference in the number of assaults against men and women psychiatrists was not statistically significant. Other studies, however, have shown that women are at greater risk than men for being assaulted. For example, Milstein's (1987) studies of psychiatric and medical house staff showed that 45% of the women residents and 35% of the men residents reported assaults. Similarly, Ruben and colleagues (1980) found that 75% of women psychiatric residents who were interviewed reported being attacked as compared with 44% of the men residents. Moreover, in Chaimowitz and Moscovitch's study (1991) of Canadian psychiatric residents, 44.8% of women and 33.3% of men were attacked.

The situations that lead to assaults against men may, similarly, lead to assaults against women. As is the case with men, women are most vulnerable to assaults when working in psychiatric emergency rooms and in acute hospital settings (Fink et al. 1991; Madden et al. 1976), although assaults also occur in outpatient settings (Dubin et al. 1988; Hatti et al. 1982). For example, a fourth-year psychiatric woman resident in a residency program was assaulted by a patient in the Veterans Administration (VA) hospital emergency room. The patient had a history of being assaultive in the past but was presently being evaluated for depression and suicidal ideation. His past diagnoses included alcohol abuse and explosive personality. At first, the resident met with the patient in the company of a security guard. During the interview, the patient gave the resident some phone numbers, including that of his mother's, so that the therapist could call people and gather additional history. The resident made the phone calls in a different room and then returned to the room with the patient, without the security guard present. She told him that she had called his mother and now was prepared to admit him to the hospital. The patient became infuriated about the fact that she had spoken to his mother. He attacked the woman resident and threw her across the room. In reviewing the incident, the staff felt that this could have happened to a man or a woman resident. There were several risk factors, including the patient's diagnoses, his history of prior violence, and the fact that the resident returned to the room with the patient without adequate security backup.

Another incident reported to the American Psychiatric Association Task Force on Clinician Safety involved a 58-year-old female psychiatrist who worked in a state hospital. She was walking up the steps on her way to a team meeting. In front of her on the steps was a 28-year-old male patient. When he was almost at the top of the stairs, he turned around and suddenly kicked her in the chest. She fell down the stairs and hit her head. She suffered two black eyes and a bruise on her chest. He later told staff that he felt that she was "messing up his brain." Although it is unknown whether the fact that the psychiatrist was a woman may have influenced the likelihood of the patient's attack, it is probable that this incident could have happened to either a man or woman clinician since it was based on a patient's delusional ideas that had nothing to do with gender.

In addition to the situations that are associated with assaults of both men and women clinicians, there are special psychodynamic, biological, and cultural considerations that may impact on a woman clinician's likelihood of being assaulted. These are discussed below.

Feelings of Vulnerability

Many authors have noted that women, in general, feel vulnerable to being attacked by men because of men's greater physical size and strength. This has been true throughout history and in many different societies (Brownmiller 1975; Russell 1975); it is also true for women clinicians. One woman resident noted that she experienced this feeling of vulnerability when she was assigned to the VA hospital. She was acutely aware that she was a woman and that nearly all of the patients were men.

Seiden (1976) pointed out that women's feelings of vulnerability are reinforced from early childhood in Western society. She noted that families are more likely to chaperone little girls than little boys. She also noted that the fear of being raped affects the psychology of all women, including those who have not been raped. Many women are encouraged to take self-defense classes or at least be trained in the basics of personal safety (Medea and Thompson 1974; Russell 1975).

Perhaps because many women are accustomed to acknowledging the fact that they are not invulnerable to attack, women clinicians use less denial in dealing with the risk of patient assault. When the Task Force on Clinician Safety met with the Committee of Residents, several women residents stated that they kept bringing up safety as an issue in their residencies. One woman said that she felt that the men residents were too "macho" to bring it up. She said that she felt comfortable admitting that she was frightened and wanted more security. Several authors have suggested that denial of the possibility of patient assaults increases the risk of being assaulted (Halleck 1989; Madden et al. 1976). It is unknown whether women's lack of denial may be protective against assaults. If the lack of denial leads to increased cautiousness, it may indeed be protective.

Lack of Authority

Levy and Harticollis (1976) pointed out that there are cultural expectations related to masculine authority. For example, male personnel have traditionally been employed to contain aggressive patients by a show of sheer physical force. The authors stated that on an inpatient unit that was staffed only by women nurses, the nurses, and also some patients, felt vaguely anxious without the presence of men, especially during the night shift.

Some women psychiatrists have reported that patients have seen them as lacking authority. One woman resident reported to the Task Force on Clinician Safety that she was asked by the staff to intervene in an incident that occurred in the dayroom on an inpatient unit. Several patients were arguing, and she told them to stop and return to their rooms. The patients ignored her. She stated that she finally had to call a male resident who went into the day room and repeated what the woman resident had said. The patients responded to the male resident's authority and dispersed to their bedrooms. One minority woman resident noted that this problem was even more difficult for her. She stated that one patient kept referring to her as a member of the housekeeping staff even though she wore her stethoscope, white coat, and name tag. When women psychiatrists feel that their authority is not being respected, they may feel even more vulnerable to being attacked by patients.

Types of Threats and Assault

Women are more likely to experience certain kinds of threats because of their gender. One kind of threat involves sexual assault. For example, a woman psychiatrist who worked in a state hospital reported to the Task Force on Clinician Safety that she was threatened by a patient who had a diagnosis of paranoid schizophrenia and a history of drug abuse. The patient stated that he was ready to leave the hospital, but the psychiatrist disagreed and told him that he was not yet ready to leave. At that point, the patient said that he would rape and kill the doctor. Subsequently, the patient apologized to the doctor. However, following the initial apology, the same scenario with the same threats occurred multiple times. The doctor stated that she was terrified and asked the clinical director to transfer the patient to another psychiatrist.

Another threatening situation involved a woman resident who worked in an inpatient setting and was approached in the hallway by a paranoid schizophrenic young man. The patient had been admitted to the hospital because he had told his treating psychiatrist that a man would be murdered, although he did not divulge the name of the victim. The resident and patient had minimal prior contact except that the therapist would smile and say hello to him when she saw him. On a particular day, however, the patient told her that she should not be frightened by the events that were about to happen. He told her that there would be many deaths but that she and he would survive and would rule the world together. After the patient was discharged from the hospital, he kept writing letters to the therapist. The letters predominantly spoke about the former patient's daily activities but also alluded to the fact that he continued to incorporate the resident in his delusions. The woman felt very frightened by these letters, which stopped after she notified the patient's outpatient psychiatrist. The woman resident wondered whether she had inadvertently acted seductively with the patient.

Some women clinicians are sexually assaulted. Chaimowitz and Moscovitch (1991) reported that one of their residents reported being sexually assaulted twice, although no details were given. In one university hospital, there was an incident involving the group psychotherapist who was a woman nurse. In the middle of a session of an inpatient group, a patient rushed over to the nurse and rubbed his hands up and down her body, including fondling her breasts. The patient was quickly removed from the room. He could not explain his behavior except to say that the nurse was pretty.

Types of Transference

Some patients are more likely to develop a maternal transference to a woman psychiatrist. At a workshop on clinician safety at the 1989 annual meeting of the American Psychiatric Association, an older woman psychiatrist recounted a frightening story of a patient's attachment to her. She noted that she had evaluated a patient before he was sent to a state prison for stabbing his ex-wife. When in prison, he stated that he thought that the psychiatrist was his mother. He stated that he intended to live with her when he was released. The woman psychiatrist asked to be notified on his release so that she could increase her security precautions. She was understandably concerned that this patient might try and find her.

Another case involved a woman resident on an acute inpatient unit who was explaining to a male schizophrenic patient that she would be taking a 1-week vacation. In his childhood, the patient had been temporarily abandoned by his mother and had been moved back and forth between his mother and a series of foster homes. He also had a history of assaulting his mother. As the resident explained her vacation plans to the patient, the patient's face took on a strange and menacing appearance. When she asked him what was going on, he said, "I'm going to beat the shit out of you." The resident became quite frightened and said in a quiet, nonthreatening voice, "Hey, remember me, I'm your friendly doctor. I'm not anyone else. I'm your doctor." The patient backed off, and she fled the room. The resident subsequently postulated that the patient had temporarily seen her as his abandoning mother.

A frightening story about the stabbing death of a 26-year-old woman social worker who reminded a patient of a friend was reported in the *National Association of Social Workers California News* (1989):

> Robbyn Panitch . . . was stabbed to death by a homeless patient on February 22, 1989, in her office at Santa Monica Mental Health Facility. Ms. Panitch was talking to her fiance on the phone at the time the assailant attacked her with a knife with a 3-inch folding blade. . . . By the time two male employees were able to disarm the patient, Robbyn had been stabbed 31 times in the face and neck. She died within

> 2 hours. When the assailant . . . was interviewed by the police, he admitted killing Robbyn because he saw her as the "Antichrist.". . . [He] believed that Panitch looked like a childhood friend he believed was the Antichrist. . . . [He] was on probation stemming from a conviction for the 1987 assault of his mother.

Some women are attacked because of other types of transference feelings. For example, a 40-year-old, white, woman psychiatrist who worked in a state hospital reported an assault to the Task Force on Clinician Safety. She walked into a nursing station, and a psychotic black woman patient suddenly attacked her and began kicking and choking her. The patient had the delusion that all white women were dating black men and, presumably, was enraged at the psychiatrist.

Pregnancy

When a woman clinician becomes pregnant, her patients, colleagues, and she herself may deal with the pregnancy in different ways that may affect the likelihood of her being assaulted. Both Lax (1969) and Benedek (1973) discussed the fact that pregnancy may evoke in patients feelings of sibling rivalry, oedipal conflicts, envy, rejection, and abandonment. Berman (1975) compared the patients of nine women psychiatrists during a period in which the therapists were pregnant with a period in which the therapists were not pregnant. She found that during pregnancy, patients, especially those who were impulsive and borderline, were more likely to act out. Paluszny and Poznanski (1971) described several cases in which patients became aggressive toward pregnant therapists. In one case, an 11-year-old boy was admitted to a hospital for repeated aggressive behavior. With treatment, his outbursts became less frequent. However, when it became obvious that his therapist was pregnant, his outbursts again became frequent. During one outburst, he hit a pregnant staff member. The authors commented on the fact that this boy had fears of abandonment and severe sibling rivalry. In a second case, they described a 38-year-old woman with breast cancer who was treated by a woman therapist who became pregnant. As the pregnancy became noticeable, the patient showed tremendous anger and hostility. She saw the baby as a new life and contrasted this with her perception of her own impending death. The authors described a third case of a 21-year-old woman who was in therapy for anxiety and depression with a pregnant therapist. The patient became angry in therapy and had the image of "twisting somebody's head off." She pictured the "somebody" as a child and thought that it might be her brother. In subsequent sessions, the patient felt angry at the therapist and had fantasies of killing both the therapist and the baby. The therapist postulated that the patient may have felt the same way when her brother was born.

There are also situations, however, in which pregnancy exerts a calming influence on patients. For example, a pregnant psychiatrist working in a hospital was evaluating an agitated schizophrenic patient. The patient started to yell at the psychiatrist but then noted her obvious pregnancy. Immediately, the patient calmed down and apologized profusely to the psychiatrist. He hoped that he had not upset her and that his yelling had not harmed the baby.

Pregnancy evokes a variety of reactions in colleagues and in staff members on an inpatient unit. The typical overt reaction of colleagues is one of overprotectiveness and oversolicitousness (Benedek 1973; Nadelson et al. 1974). Leibenluft (1984) studied several inpatient units where the staff seemed much more concerned with protecting the pregnant women than the women did. When Leibenluft interviewed pregnant clinicians, they stated that safety was not their primary concern but that they were comfortable with peripheral involvement in seclusion procedures and were appreciative of staff assignments that permitted them to avoid direct interaction with potentially violent patients. In contrast, all but one of the nonpregnant staff began their interviews with Leibenluft by talking of the need to protect pregnant women from violent patients. She also pointed out that there is reluctance by some staff to express anger to a pregnant staff member. For example, on one unit that she studied, a staff member said, "How can you get angry at a pregnant woman?" Two staff members had the fantasy that a direct expression of their anger would cause a premature delivery. Several staff members said they did not want to ruin a woman's feelings of happiness about being pregnant by being angry. This overprotectiveness and oversolicitousness may decrease the risk of women getting assaulted if staff intervene quickly in potentially assaultive episodes.

Other reactions, however, have also been described. Benedek (1973) pointed out that many of the staff tend to deny the fact of a pregnancy, especially during the early stages. Leibenluft (1984), Butts and Cavenar (1979), and Auchincloss (1982) discussed the negative feelings toward pregnant therapists, including envy, jealousy, anxiety about impending separation, and resentment about the needed staffing changes. It is possible that these feelings of denial and negative feelings could lead to a staff's underreactions to a potentially dangerous situation involving a pregnant therapist on an inpatient unit or in a psychiatric emergency room.

Pregnancy also evokes a variety of reactions in pregnant women themselves. As Nadelson and colleagues (1974) pointed out, during pregnancy, clinicians experience increased physical and emotional vulnerability. Paluszny and Poznanski (1971) and Baum and Herring (1975) noted that pregnant women experience fatigue and may be more distractible because of their preoccupation with thoughts of the baby. Further, as noted by Nadelson and colleagues (1974), some women may react to the changes during their pregnancy by denying their needs and taking on more work to prove their capabilities. Some women feel that having allowances made for them during their pregnancy makes them feel that being a woman means being an inadequate physician or therapist. One example of this denial was displayed by a woman psychiatrist who during her two pregnancies worked on a locked inpatient unit that treated the most violent patients in the hospital. She denied that she was at risk at all. She told residents that she felt perfectly safe during her pregnancies working on that unit and, in fact, how she had worked until the day before her delivery. Other women are more aware of their vulnerabilities during pregnancy and ask not to be assigned to inpatient units with violent patients. Even those women who might not request extra security measures for themselves are more likely to request extra security to protect an unborn baby. Nadelson and colleagues (1974) suggested that perhaps pregnant women should not be assigned to work with violent patients. Baum and Herring (1975) discussed the importance of flexibility in residency programs for pregnant residents.

Psychological Reactions After an Assault

The psychological effects of an assault on a clinician can be devastating. This is true for both men and women. Women can develop symptoms of posttraumatic stress disorder. For example, one woman resident who was interviewed stated that after she was assaulted, she had nightmares, intrusive images, and crying spells. She also had difficulty concentrating and was fearful of taking further night call. Assaults can also affect family members. For example, one woman noted that her children were upset after she was assaulted. She said that even at the present time her children ask her when she returns from work, "Are you okay? Did you get hurt today?" After an assault, women clinicians are sometimes embarrassed and have concerns that others may blame them. This is similar to what is experienced by some rape victims (Binder 1981). These reactions may lead to underreporting of assaults (Lion et al. 1981). It is important that colleagues and supervisors who review assaults with clinicians not blame the victim when making suggestions or discussing what might have been done differently.

Conclusions

Female as well as male clinicians are assaulted by patients. In general, women acknowledge that they feel vulnerable to assault and that this may lead to increased cautiousness. However, women also experience a perceived lack of authority that may make them more vulnerable. Further, women are more likely than men to have certain unique types of threats, assaults, and transferences directed toward them. These transferences may make them more vulnerable to attack. Pregnancy of clinicians may provoke assaults or conversely protect women from assaults. Vulnerability during pregnancy may be related to feelings evoked in patients, in colleagues, and in the woman herself. There is a need to gather more information about the incidence and risk factors related to assaults against women and to devise further strategies for prevention.

References

Auchincloss EL: Conflict among psychiatric residents in response to pregnancy. Am J Psychiatry 139:818–821, 1982

Baum DE, Herring C: The pregnant psychotherapist in training: some preliminary findings and impressions. Am J Psychiatry 132:419–422, 1975

Benedek E: The fourth world of the pregnant therapist. J Am Med Wom Assoc 28:365–368, 1973

Berman E: Acting out as a response to the psychiatrist's pregnancy. J Am Med Wom Assoc 30:456–458, 1975

Binder RL: Why women don't report sexual assault. J Clin Psychiatry 42:437–438, 1981

Brownmiller S: Against Our Will: Men, Women and Rape. New York, Simon & Schuster, 1975

Butts NT, Cavenar JO Jr: Colleagues' responses to the pregnant psychiatric resident. Am J Psychiatry 136:1587–1589, 1979

Carmel H, Hunter M: Staff injuries from inpatient violence. Hosp Community Psychiatry 40:41–46, 1989

Chaimowitz GA, Moscovitch A: Patient assaults against psychiatric residents: the Canadian experience. Can J Psychiatry 36:107–111, 1991

Dubin WR, Wilson SJ, Mercer C: Assaults against psychiatrists in outpatient settings. J Clin Psychiatry 49:410–419, 1988

Fink DL, Dubin W, Shoyer B: A study of assaults against psychiatric residents. Academic Psychiatry 15:94–99, 1991

Halleck SI: When residents are victims of violence. Academic Psychiatry 13:113–115, 1989

Hatti S, Dubin WR, Weiss KJ: A study of circumstances surrounding patient assaults on psychiatrists. Hosp Community Psychiatry 33:660–661, 1982

Lax RE: Some considerations about transference and countertransference manifestations evoked by the analyst's pregnancy. Am J Psychoanal 50:363–372, 1969

Leibenluft E: Staff responses to the pregnancy of a therapist on an inpatient unit. Hosp Community Psychiatry 35:1033–1036, 1984

Levy P, Harticollis P: Nursing aides and patient violence. Am J Psychiatry 133:429–431, 1976

Lion RJ, Snyder W, Merrill GL: Underreporting of assaults in a state hospital. Hosp Community Psychiatry 32:497–498, 1981

Madden DJ, Lion JR, Penna MW: Assaults on psychiatrists by patients. Am J Psychiatry 133:422–425, 1976

Medea A, Thompson K: Against Rape. New York, Farrar, Straus & Giroux, 1974

Milstein V: Patient assaults on residents. Indiana Medicine 80:753–755, 1987

Nadelson C, Notman M, Arons E, et al: The pregnant therapist. Am J Psychiatry 131:1107–1111, 1974

National Association of Social Workers California News, Vol 15, No 7, April 1989

Paluszny M, Poznanski E: Reactions of patients during pregnancy of the psychotherapist. Child Psychiatry Hum Dev 4:266–274, 1971

Ruben I, Wolkon G, Yamamoto J: Physical attacks on psychiatric residents by patients. J Nerv Ment Dis 168:243–245, 1980

Russell DE: The Politics of Rape. New York, Stein & Day, 1975

Seiden AM: Overview: research on the psychology of women, I: gender differences and sexual and reproductive life. Am J Psychiatry 133:995–1007, 1976

Tardiff K, Maurice WL: The care of violent patients by psychiatrists. Canadian Psychiatric Association Journal 22:83–86, 1977

Whitman RM, Armao BB, Dent OB: Assault on the therapist. Am J Psychiatry 133:426–429, 1976

Chapter 4

Violence and Psychiatric Residency

David Fink, M.D.

Despite a rising tide of violence in contemporary society, there has been little study of the risks of violence as a part of medical practice. Concern about violence predictably increases in the wake of the most extreme and occasionally tragic incidents in which a physician is attacked or killed. The organized response to those tragedies that capture professional and public attention, however, has been meager. There has been no large-scale systematic study of violence against physicians.

Although available literature suggests that psychiatrists in their work with mentally ill patients face a particularly high risk of assault, other physicians are in no way immune. The recent murder of Dr. Katheryn Hinnant, a pathologist at Bellevue Hospital in New York City, is a worst-case scenario in which a physician not directly involved in an individual patient's care was violently assaulted. The murder occurred on a weekend in an unsecured part of the hospital. Although shock, fear, anger, and concern were ubiquitous among Bellevue staff following the incident, so was a sense of resignation and acceptance of the fact of violence as a part of clinical practice. An article from *American Medical News* (Somerville 1989) revealed this resignation to violence:

> In the emergency room you are as likely to be punched as thanked . . . sometimes it is more than a fist that threatens the physicians, however.

Portions of this chapter were adapted from Fink D, Shoyer B, Dubin WR: "A Study of Assaults Against Psychiatric Residents." *Academic Psychiatry* 15:94–99, 1991.

> I had a patient pull a knife on me. . . . We're endangering our lives by coming to work. It adds to the incredible stress of working here.

Clearly, all physicians are exposed to some risk during practice. Residents, in particular, may face greater risks because they characteristically spend the greatest number of hours in the hospital and work during the least secured times, nights and weekends. Although anecdotal reports support the increased risk and exposure for trainees, formal study of dangerousness during training across specialty areas in medicine is meager. In the only available study of violence against medical residents that surveyed trainees from all fields of medicine, Levin (1987) surveyed residents in training in California for information on acts of violence or attempted violence against residents or medical personnel. Levin's survey followed the murders of two residents and the beating of a medical student. Of the 200 residents who responded, 24% said they or fellow staff members had been assaulted. In this survey, knives or guns were involved in 40% of the attacks. Levin found that the emergency room and admitting area were the most common settings for violence and attempted violence, accounting for about one-third of all acts. Levin also found, however, that half of all attacks occurred in other areas of the hospital, including wards, patient rooms, resident call rooms, and private offices. This preliminary study indicates that a quarter of all residents in this index program were victims of violence during training. Although Levin identified a considerable risk, the study is limited in that it does not assess differences across specialty areas. Additionally, the restriction to a single residency program prohibits generalization of the findings to risks of violence for residents in general.

At the Indiana University School of Medicine, Milstein (1987) compared the rate of assaults among psychiatric and medical residents within the Indiana training program. Of the 33 psychiatric residents and 117 medical residents surveyed, 39% of the psychiatric residents, but only 16% of the medical residents, were assaulted. In both groups, the percentage of trainees reporting assaults increased with each postgraduate year. In both groups, a larger proportion of female residents reported assaults than male residents: 45% female to 35% male in psychiatry and 23% female to 14% male in medicine. Although Levin's (1987) and Milstein's (1987) work suggests a considerable risk of violence for residents in all areas of training, the incidence of acts of violence perpetrated against residents in general has not been defined and awaits a large-scale multicenter incidence study.

As a specialty, psychiatry has looked more closely at issues of violence than have other branches of medicine. Several large surveys have defined the career risk of assault against a psychiatrist to be in the range of 40%–50% (Madden et al. 1976; Milstein 1987). Further, surveys that have included psychiatric residents have demonstrated that psychiatric residents have a higher rate of assault than their more senior colleagues. Of the 115 psychiatrists surveyed by Madden and colleagues, 65% of the respondents who had been assaulted were residents at the time of the assault. In a study of violence against psychiatrists at Atascadero State Hospital in California, Carmel and Hunter (1990) found that younger psychiatrists and psychiatrists more recently out of residency were subject to a greater number of assaults.

Ruben and colleagues (1980) were the first to look independently at the risk of violence for psychiatric residents. In their survey of 31 second- and third-year residents in training at the University of Southern California Medical Center, they found that 48% of the respondents had been attacked at least once during training. The most common explanation given by the residents for the attacks was that they had frustrated the patient. All but two of the attacks occurred with psychotic patients not previously known to the resident. Attacks occurred on all clinical psychiatric services. Ruben and colleagues attempted to define characteristics of those assaulted and suggested that residents who were highly irritable, who speak up when angry, and who are likely to fight when faced with a physically threatening situation were more likely to be assaulted than those who did not have these attributes.

Gray (1989) surveyed 73 psychiatry residents at all levels of training within the same program and found an assault rate of 54%. Relative risks of assault were slightly higher in female, nonwhite, and younger residents, but the differences were not statistically significant. The child and adolescent services, followed by the emergency service, were the sites of highest risk. The outpatient service had the lowest risk of assault. The most common assailant was a white, psychotic, young, adult male previously unknown to the resident. The most common form of attack was being struck with fists or kicked. Most assaults did not result in serious physical injury. For example, in one serious assault, a resident was threatened with a knife; in another, a resident was the victim of an attempted strangulation. Although the stability of the rate of assault, within this one program over the course of a decade, identifies an alarmingly high rate of patient-resident violence, neither the studies by Ruben and colleagues (1980) nor the study by Gray allow generalization to residents in other settings. It remains unclear to what extent these high assault rates reflect risks specific to the training experience at the University of Southern California.

Two studies have attempted to expand on these preliminary findings and more broadly define the risks of violence against psychiatric residents. Chaimowitz and Moscovitch (1991) surveyed all the members in training of the Canadian Psychiatric Association. Of the 136 (64.5%) respondents, 40% indicated that they had been assaulted by a patient at least once. Of the female residents, 45% had been assaulted compared with 33% of the male residents. Although the majority were assaulted once (60.4%), 31% were assaulted twice, and 8% were assaulted three or more times. Of those assaulted, 25% felt that the incident was due to an error on their part, 45% felt it was part of the risk of psychiatric practice, 51% felt that the attack was totally unpredictable, and 32% felt the assault was related to unsafe facilities. Although half of the residents reported that they had received some training in dealing with violent patients, only a quarter felt that they had been adequately trained. Chaimowitz and Moscovitch were the first to measure rates of violence against residents across a wide range of clinical sites and training programs. The assault rate of 40% during the course of a 4-year residency program is comparable to the career rate of assaults for psychiatrists found in other studies (Madden et al. 1976; Milstein 1987) and confirms that residency training is a time of particularly high risk for assault.

A study by Fink and colleagues (1991) corroborated Chaimowitz and Moscovitch's (1991) findings and indicated that this high rate of violence is not specific to the Canadian training experience. Fink and colleagues surveyed all 333 psychiatric residents in training in the state of Pennsylvania. Of the 155 (46%) respondents, 41% had been assaulted and 48% had been threatened during training. A small group of residents (10%) were assaulted multiple times. The Pennsylvania study, in an effort to refine the evaluation of dangerousness, defined subtypes of assaults and threats. Assaults were divided into three categories based on the degree of physician harm incurred during the incident. Serious assaults were defined as assaults that required medical attention (e.g., stabbing, biting, or blows to the head resulting in concussion). Moderate assaults were defined as incidents characterized by aggressive intent in which some physical contact was made (e.g., scratches, pokes, shoves, or being hit with objects or fists). Assaults with potential for harm were defined as actions with aggressive intent in which no physical contact was made; these included thrown objects and attempted but unsuccessful assaults with weapons. Of the assaults, 69% were moderate, 53% had potential for harm, and 3% were serious. A total of 187 assaults was reported by 63 residents. Threats were similarly categorized into written threats, verbal threats face to face, verbal threats over the phone, and other types of threats. Of 318 threats made to 74 residents, 60% were face to face, and 25% were made over the phone. Other types of threats and written threats occurred in 13% and 2% of the cases, respectively. Although no correlation was found between rates of threats or assaults and the age or sex of the residents, there was a strong correlation between the site of clinical activity and rates of violence. The majority of threats or assaults occurred on the inpatient unit (56%) or in the psychiatric emergency room (31%). In addition, the majority of the incidents of violence occurred during night call and weekends, a time of relatively low structure and decreased staff availability. The other time of high risk for threats and assaults was during restraint procedures and involuntary commitments.

The most common reasons for the assault or threat given by the residents were refusing to meet a patient's request (59%), setting a limit (44%), making a comment unfavorably received (29%), not setting enough limits (14%), and forcing a patient to take a medication (14%). Although most of the residents suggested that the incident was a random and unpredictable event, approximately half indicated that they had either a moderate or a strong sense of dangerousness before the threat or assault. This contradiction minimizes the role of the resident in the interaction. Very few respondents felt that interpersonal factors or transference or countertransference forces played a role in the violent event. Of the respondents, 11% felt that transference factors were important triggers to the violent episode, 6% implicated troubling material being dealt with in psychotherapy, and 1% indicated that projection was involved in the incident. Similarly, only 7% felt that fear of the patient or projected dislike of the patient by the resident played a role.

In contrast, other studies identified a much greater interpersonal role in incidents of violence. Ruben and colleagues (1980) suggested that more "irritable" residents were more frequently assaulted. Chaimowitz and Moscovitch (1991) found that 25% of the residents identified an error on their part that may have sparked a violent response. Madden and colleagues (1976) found that 55% of psychiatrists had evidence before the session of the assault that the patient was dangerous, and 53% felt that they may have acted in a provocative manner. Both Fink and colleagues (1991) and Chaimowitz and Moscovitch surveyed residents' responses to violence in terms of reporting to supervisors or the penal or legal systems. Fink and colleagues found that 67% of the residents reported an episode of threat or assault to a supervisor, 30% reported to a medical or residency director, and 6% reported an assault to a law enforcement agency. In the Canadian group (Chaimowitz and Moscovitch 1991), 74% of the assaults were reported to an administrator. Chaimowitz and Moscovitch explored residents' attitudes about reporting acts of violence that might account for the 26% of residents who failed to report acts of aggression to supervisors and might contribute to a more general tendency toward underreporting of assaults. Investigators found an array of concerns and reasons for underreporting among their survey group: 1) no clear reporting process; 2) lack of administrative support; 3) shame, guilt, and denial of the importance of the event; 4) fear of scrutiny; 5) staff members' being blamed for lack of caution and anticipation; 6) denial on the part of other staff since the event is so close to home; 7) attitudes among staff that assaults are normal and a part of the job; or 8) attitudes among staff that attempts at change are futile. Fink and colleagues found similar concerns about the reporting process among the Pennsylvania residents. Many residents expressed frustrations at the lack of an available process for reporting violent episodes. Many feared being blamed or stigmatized for violence done against them.

The available studies confirm that a substantial percentage, approximately 40%, of psychiatric residents will be assaulted at least once during the course of a 4-year residency (Chaimowitz and Moscovitch 1991; Fink et al. 1991; Gray 1989; Ruben et al. 1980). The data contradict the view that acts of violence are extremely rare and therefore do not warrant administrative attention. Violence against residents cannot be considered as an occasional and acceptable risk of training. Studies by Chaimowitz and Moscovitch and Fink and colleagues suggested that denial plays a significant role in the residents' approach to the potentially violent patient, as well as in the attitudes of the supervising staff and residency directors.

Denial of dangerousness and the minimalizing of risks of violence are reflected in the meager amount of residency training time dedicated to the understanding of aggression and work with the violent patient. The two studies that explored the extent of training in work with violent patients revealed an insufficient training experience in most cases. Of the Pennsylvania residents, 122 (79%) had received some training in managing violent patients (Fink et al. 1991). The amount of training time ranged from 1 to 10 hours, with a mean of 3 hours during the course of a residency. Typical training consisted of 2 hours of classroom time and 1.5 hours of preceptorial time. In contrast, residents reported an average of 8 hours of didactic classroom time and 7 hours of preceptorial time in the study of the suicidal patient. Four times as many hours are spent in learning about suicide in contrast to violence or homicide. Chaimowitz and Moscovitch (1991) noted that issues of aggression receive little attention; 50% of the respondents had received some training in dealing with violent patients, but only 25% felt that they had been adequately trained. In this latter group, the residents perceived themselves as the most poorly trained when compared with nurses and staff psychiatrists.

In a commentary exploring violence against residents, Halleck (1989) echoed the areas of greatest concern voiced by residents in the Canadian and Pennsylvania studies. The first area of concern pertained to the establishment of a safe treatment setting, particularly in terms of the physical structure of the interview room, entrances and exits, access to help, and warning systems. The second area addressed adequate training and preparation of residents before exposure to difficult and potentially dangerous clinical situations.

> Psychiatric training programs traditionally place their least experienced doctors in the most difficult treatment situations. . . . Recent medical graduates in nonpsychiatric specialties begin their first year of training with a reasonable degree of experience in managing physical aspects of illness. Beginning psychiatric residents, however, have learned very little about managing psychiatric patients. Until they have been tutored, precepted, and had the chance to watch others handle difficult situations many times over or unless a more advanced resident or attending is physically present, they should never be allowed to

manage the most difficult patients in the most difficult situations in psychiatry. (Halleck 1989, p. 114)

Currently, residents perceive themselves as unprepared and undertrained for interactions with violently or potentially violent patients; training is felt to be insufficient. Several studies clearly indicate that training in aggression management can be effectively taught and that this can result in a decrease in the incidence of assaults (Infantino and Musingo 1985; Maier 1986). Halleck (1989) proposed a supervisory and on-site preceptorial experience for residents to learn approaches to work with aggressive patients. A sample curriculum for residency training in aggression management compiled by the American Psychiatric Association Task Force on Clinician Safety (Dubin and Lion 1992) elucidated the knowledge base about aggression with which all residents should be familiar. All residents should receive instruction in the biological, sociological, and psychological antecedents of violence. Attention should be paid to evaluating violent patients, with particular focus on differential diagnosis of toxic metabolic states and organic mental disorders. The response to the agitated, violent, or threatening patient should be considered across several domains. Residents should receive instruction in verbal and behavioral approaches to the violent patient. Attention should be paid to paraverbal communications and interactions that might stabilize the escalating patient. The pharmacologic management of the violent patient should be taught. Residents should be familiar both with both appropriate standards for seclusion and restraint and with restraint techniques. Residents should become familiar with the psychodynamic processes that are commonly activated and play a part in aggression and acts of violence, including the roles of projection and displacement and how to work with these defenses.

Psychiatry has looked more closely at risks of practice and rates of violence against clinicians than all other branches of medicine. Despite this consideration, however, the study of aggression in the clinical setting is in its infancy. As Madden and colleagues (1976) and Lion and Pasternak (1973) have pointed out, denial of dangerousness is a ubiquitous defense and compounds the difficulty of carrying out large-scale studies of violence. Denial must not result in the minimalization of this considerable risk to clinicians or in undermining the implementation of sensible educational and administrative policy guidelines. Matters of clinical safety can be taught and should be addressed as an essential part of all residency training. Beyond classroom and preceptorial experiences focused on work with violent patients, all residencies should have a procedure in place to monitor and follow up on acts of violence that involve trainees. Violence is a pervasive social concern and one that increasingly enters the domain of medical and psychiatric practice. Measures must be taken to minimize the risk for clinicians and to educate clinicians in how to manage violence when it occurs.

References

Carmel H, Hunter M: Psychiatrists injured by patient attack. Paper presented at the annual meeting of the American Academy of Psychiatry and the Law, San Diego, California, October 27, 1990

Chaimowitz GA, Moscovitch A: Patient assaults against psychiatric residents: the Canadian experience. Can J Psychiatry 36:107–111, 1991

Dubin WR, Lion JR (eds): Clinician Safety: Report of the American Psychiatric Association Task Force on Clinician Safety. Washington, DC, American Psychiatric Association, 1992

Fink D, Shoyer B, Dubin WR: Study of assaults against psychiatric residents. Academic Psychiatry 15:94–99, 1991

Gray GE: Assaults by patients against psychiatric residents at a public psychiatric hospital. Academic Psychiatry 13:81–85, 1989

Halleck SI: When residents are victims of violence. Academic Psychiatry 13:113–115, 1989

Infantino JA, Musingo SY: Assaults and injuries among staff with and without training in aggression control techniques. Hosp Community Psychiatry 36:1312–1314, 1985

Levin S: American Medical News, July 3, 1987

Lion J, Pasternak SA: Countertransference reactions to violent patients. Am J Psychiatry 130:207–210, 1973

Madden DJ, Lion JR, Penna MW: Assaults on psychiatrists by patients. Am J Psychiatry 133:422–425, 1976

Maier GJ: Relationship security: the dynamics of keepers and kept. J Forensic Sci 31:603–608, 1986

Milstein V: Patient assaults on residents. Indiana Medicine 80:753–755, 1987

Ruben I, Wolkon G, Yamamoto J: Physical attacks on psychiatric residents by patients. J Nerv Ment Dis 168:243–245, 1980

Somerville J: Violence to MDs more widespread than thought. American Medical News, February 10, 1989

Chapter 5

Verbal Threats Against Clinicians

John R. Lion, M.D.

In the course of my work with violent patients, I have been occasionally asked to intervene or offer suggestions regarding a patient who has made a verbal threat against a mental health professional. These consultations have been requested several times a year, and there have been sufficient similarities in the circumstances of the threats to warrant the description that follows in this chapter. At the outset, it is my impression that threats are actually quite common in psychotherapeutic work, particularly on hospital wards. They also occur in outpatient and in private practice settings, where therapy can be considerably more intense.

Yet there is sparse literature on the specific topic of threats (as opposed to assaults) in clinical practice. More than 20 years ago, MacDonald (1967) studied 100 patients who had made homicidal threats and determined after a 5-year follow-up that four patients had committed suicide and three others homicide; this article remains an important clinical study demonstrating the vector problem of assessing risk of violence. Bernstein (1981) surveyed a sample of therapists in San Diego, California, and found that 35% of the group had been threatened. Billowitz and Pendleton (1988) published an article on the intervention strategies used to deal with a threatening patient in a hospital setting.

I have generally found that denial is the principal defense utilized in dealing with violent threats. Indeed, when asked to intervene in a situation in which there has been a verbal threat, I am, more often than not, apt to find the threat to be old or repetitive. In some cases, the patient has made threats for weeks or months and the therapist and staff have made only feeble attempts to cope with it. When the situations are viewed retrospectively, all become aware of their resistance to grapple with what is obviously a serious and escalating problem; yet strong intragroup forces mitigate against the mobilizing of decisive action.

> *Case A.* A mental health center staff asked for guidance concerning threats made on two members of their staff by a patient who had been in treatment for several years. A young man diagnosed as having a severe impulse character disorder developed paranoid ideation about a female psychologist and a male psychiatrist who were coleaders of the group therapy in which the patient was enrolled. Because the patient was so stormy in the sessions, both leaders worked individually with him for a while to no avail. The patient continued to be argumentative, volatile, and accusatory, stating that no one cared or could help him. Subsequently, he began phoning the psychologist and leaving threatening messages on her answering machine. He spoke of "getting her" and "taking care she would not work any more." He also came to the clinic and boldly demanded to see the psychiatrist, who then confronted the patient and asked him to leave the premises. The patient was verbally abusive and frightening. However, months elapsed before the psychologist asked the police for assistance regarding the patient's harassment of her. When I met with the staff, their primary concern was whether reporting him to the police would lead him to become retributive and what their obligation was to the patient.

This case illustrates the principle of denial but more starkly shows how chronic the threats were. Actually, the threats dated back almost a year before I was informed about them. This delay always raises the interesting question of what threshold event finally catalyzes the request for help. In the field of family violence, it has long been observed that by the time violence reaches public awareness, tacit acceptance has been deeply ingrained with the family structure. I have been impressed with not only the power of the threat but how the threat contains cohesive force for a whole staff. Clearly, the threats produced a spirit of camaraderie and mission, giving members of the clinic a strange, but important, sense of purpose. This aspect of the threat cannot be underscored enough: violence and the threat of violence, if long standing, serve an important group process function and cannot be easily eliminated, even if common sense dictates a clear solution. In this case, it was obvious that the psychologist had evidence (tape recordings) to prosecute the patient. But such evidence was not used, and more complex dynamics emerged as my familiarity with the case increased.

For instance, the psychologist was unmarried, as was the patient; some of the latter's messages had romantic overtones with fantasies of matrimony. Staff were split on their management of the patient, some believing him to be dangerous, others viewing him as a nuisance. No attempt was made to assess clinically his potential for harm on the basis of past history (he had been violent and been incarcerated) or to determine how limits might be set on his behavior. Indeed, the entire question of whether the clinic could or even should have ever handled him was never reviewed.

Such omissions in assessment seem outrageous and, at first glance, would appear to reflect the practice of people with little clinical training. But this was not the case. The clinic in fact had very qualified and trained personnel who were intuitive and sensitive. I have often seen this with staff who encounter and grapple with threats; far from being negligent or indifferent, personnel are often well-trained individuals who bend over backward to be fair, reasonable, and persevering. Indeed, the persistent reasonableness of their responses in the face of danger may be pathological in and of itself.

Additionally, in this example, the patient actually made a complaint against the psychologist's professional board and challenged both her competence and her propriety. This led to a formal review by the licensing board. The psychologist was cleared, of course, but I expected far more anger at this considerable inconvenience than was evident from my discussion with her. The puzzling absence of anger is also a feature of the second case. There is, in both cases, a bizarre fascination with the threatening person and a pathological tolerance of the situation.

Case B. An analytically trained psychiatrist in a large metropolitan area phoned me for consultation regarding a private patient of his who was leaving threatening messages on his answering machine. The therapist had seen the man for several years and currently saw him twice weekly. The therapist was calm in his account of the threats and professed wonder about them rather than alarm. The threats were ominous-sounding laughter and messages to the effect that he "should beware." The therapist did not talk to the patient about the threats, and I learned that the therapist was going on vacation. When he returned, he found that the patient had repeatedly left more threats on the answering machine. The seeming indifference of the therapist was noteworthy. Obviously, he must have cared sufficiently to phone me long distance. The lack of affect was an important clue, and the case demonstrates a recurring issue in the matter of threats—the failure or inability to monitor the transference. I discovered in further talks with the therapist that his patient occasionally entered the office and playfully made a strangle-like gesture to the therapist as he passed by him to take his seat. This had somehow not been taken up in the context of the therapy.

Therapists who treat more primitive character disorders or paranoid or psychotic patients run a certain risk as closeness develops, a risk that must be continuously assessed and dealt with. But the very feeling and behaviors that signal the risk must be carefully scrutinized. More subtle actions such as the patient's moving his chair back slightly or defensive posturing or tardiness occurring late in the course of therapy should alert the clinician to the problem of the transference. As to the clinical aloofness that may characterize the therapist's manner, it may serve as a deterrent to the fruitful discussion of transference and, in my experience, may even exacerbate a negative one in which the therapist is viewed as cold and cruel, deserving of a threat. Whereas most clinicians understand that the overidealization of a borderline patient may easily turn to disdain and even ragefulness, it is less well recognized that the seeming detachment of a patient may in time change into anger. This is particularly true of more schizoid or schizotypal patients, who appear controlled or cautious in therapy, yet may harbor underlying hostility at a therapist whom they feel has too intimate a knowledge of them and controls them.

Case C. A psychiatric trainee presented the case of a young schizophrenic patient whose pathology he found quite chronic. The trainee was, nonetheless, encouraged by the senior staff to treat the patient psychotherapeutically to assess the latter's capacity for improvement. The trainee met several times a week with the patient. In time, the patient showed increasing affect and became more verbal; he also began to utter threats directed at both the trainee and at the president of the United States. This threat required that the Secret Service be called to assess the patient's dangerousness.

Although other factors played a role in this case, including possible hypomanic activation with the use of antidepressant medication, it was felt by the trainee and his supervisor that transference had gotten out of hand and that the threats represented, in large measure, the patient's psychotic attempts to halt further intimacy. Staff were surprised by the seemingly explosive blossoming of the transference. Some threats on clinicians may arise precipitously but nevertheless reflect ongoing psychodynamic processes that can be satisfactorily elucidated; threats are not random events. In this case, the patient seemed overloaded with affectively laden issues through individual and family therapy sessions. His public threats led to the notification of the Secret Service and further detainment in the hospital. The trainee was frightened of the threats but finally confronted the patient and explored the transference. Thereafter, the threats subsided.

Case D. A young borderline male was in private therapy with a clinician on a twice-weekly basis. The treatment proceeded well, and the patient appeared grateful, but over the second year of therapy he began to express some anger and told the therapist that he had applied for a gun permit for his home. The therapist did not discuss this fact nor did he confront the patient's continued anger at him until the patient mentioned, while paying his bill to the office secretary, that he thought about killing the therapist. The secretary immediately informed a member of the group practice, who urgently confronted his colleague, suggesting immediate hospitalization for the patient. This was accomplished. However, the therapist felt bad about the deterioration of treatment and visited the patient in the hospital until he was exhorted to stop by his colleagues. Thereafter, the patient was transferred to another therapist.

This case illustrates an unmonitored transference and the difficulty a therapist can have with separation. He and the patient had worked together for a long time, and he was proud of the progress the patient had made. No health practitioner is free of such pride, but the positive gains made in this client's psychotherapy must be balanced with a realization of an intense transference that the patient had focused on the therapist. Such transference can be dangerous. Potentially violent borderline or paranoid individuals should be seen in a more public place where there are other staff and where the institutional ambience serves to dilute what may otherwise be a threatening experience.

Case E. Two senior clinicians from an outpatient clinic called to discuss what decision their facility should make about a situation involving a young, borderline, assaultive female patient who was

> threatening to kill her husband. She had also threatened the clinic staff. They described how difficult the patient was, how tenuous their treatment strategy was, and how much trouble she had caused for the clinic. They were quite upset about their legal responsibility to the spouse.

I would not wish to propose that every negative reaction to a threatening or violent patient represents undetected transference. Some patients may simply be too volatile and not treatable in an outpatient setting. A second conversation with the above clinicians convinced all of us that this patient probably needed inpatient care, although it appeared that she was unlikely to accept this idea. Thus, discharge from the clinic might be in order. But the doctors brought up the issue of their duty toward the patient, and I found myself again counseling against excessive "patience and understanding" with a patient.

I have often found myself in the position of telling a clinician or staff that they should not be treating the threatening patient and that the patient should go elsewhere. Rejoinders to such advice usually are couched in quasi-ethical terms ("But he's a patient!"). Beyond care for an acutely homicidal or suicidal patient, a clinician can disengage from a patient, particularly when the situation poses some danger for the therapist. But disengagement is often the most difficult task. To some extent, the clinical problem may be compared to the problem of marital separation when two parties are locked together in a pathological relationship.

In Case A, this was certainly the case when it took much effort to get the psychologist to press legal charges against the patient and terminate contact. Actually, the police proved helpful in this venture by preventing the therapist from seeing or talking to the patient. Law officers and attorneys are often more useful in helping clinicians distance themselves from unpalatable clinical situations than fellow mental health professionals. This may be due to their experience with the problem of terminating relationships and their ability intuitively to understand the fact that the perpetuation of such relationships may endanger each party. One can speculate that the morbidity and mortality of the mental health profession, in terms of depression, stems from the tendency to internalize aggression; an effect of such internalization is an inability to be directly angry with patients. Mental health professionals are often surprisingly free of hostile feelings at the very patients who threaten or even assault them.

Case F. A young male inpatient returned from a night's leave in an intoxicated and rageful state. He was asked to go to bed but became violent, destroying furniture on the ward and threatening staff, including the psychiatrist on call. The threats consisted of shouts of, "I'm gonna get you," and continued until the patient was detained by the hospital police and committed to a state facility. Staff met with me after the incident to discuss their adamant request for better security and the installation of panic alarms on the ward. The question arose as to whether or not to press charges against the patient for the destruction of property. No one wished to do this. Further, the psychiatrist bristled at all suggestions or attempts to discuss the incident.

The incident was clearly a frightening one for all parties involved, yet the magnitude of the fear was not coupled with anger at the patient. Again, affect appeared to be handled by demands for physical safety. After my discussions, some staff, including the psychiatrist, were able to verbalize the fear that pressing charges might induce the patient to become vindictive. Other staff members did not wish to get involved, and still others saw the pressing of legal charges against a psychiatric patient, albeit a nonpsychotic one, as hopeless. The police were more optimistic and offered to help, but, in the end, nothing was done.

Retributive and retaliatory fears represent one of the biggest obstacles to the handling of threats by staff and, usually, are the manifestation of anger on the part of staff—anger that is handled by projection. In other writings (Lion 1987; Lion and Pasternak 1973; Lion and Reid 1983), I have described how such displaced anger hinders the acceptance of the clinician's own rage. Even in the case of threats that are well documented by the presence of witnesses or tape recordings, and where legal action could be taken, few clinicians opt for prosecution. The issue of prosecution for violent patients is a fascinating one that has been described elsewhere (Appelbaum and Appelbaum, Chapter 11, this volume; Hoge and Gutheil 1987). It is interesting to note that the mere discussion of the option to prosecute often catalyzes a therapeutic outpouring of feelings concerning the patient. When staff members recognize that they are angry with a patient, they are usually in a better position to handle the situation.

Direct confrontation is often useful for those who are threatened. I often urge clinicians to tell patients that they (the patients) are frightening. Comments such as "You're scaring me with your threats" or queries such as "Why do you have to go around scaring me and others with your threats—is this the only way you can relate to people—to be scary?" are critical therapeutic messages to be made. Unfortunately, I invariably encounter skepticism, and clinicians reply that they feel uncomfortable telling a patient that they are frightened; such an admission, they state, may only show the patient how powerful he or she is and worsen a bad situation. However, threats are the means by which patients establish control and repudiate those near them. Threats put a wedge in the therapeutic relationship. Threats repel. The proper strategy, then, is to acknowledge the behavior on the patient's part by the appropriate interpretation by the therapist. If the patient hears that the threats are indeed producing the desired distance, the patient may stop. If everyone pretends that the threats are having no effect, the patient may escalate the threats.

If there exists an alliance with the patient, the second set of interpretative statements can be made, such as "Why do you go around threatening and alienating people?" or "Do you have any positive feelings about our therapy—about being in this hospital?" Such exploration may, of course, be untenable with disturbed patients who are not firmly "seated" in therapy, and I do not wish to undermine my earlier suggestion that the patients who threaten be considered for termination of treatment. The therapist may try to clarify the meaning of the threat, but failure of the patient to respond to reasonable intervention and continued threats are considerations for termination of therapy. I often ask staff how they would handle the patient if the person were not a psychiatric patient but simply a visitor or a person on the street. The reply is almost universally one of rejection.

Case G. A psychiatric resident related to me that a patient he had seen in the emergency room and committed to a state hospital had muttered a threat as he was taken out the door by the attendants. The resident felt anxious about the threat and wanted to know what the chances were of having something happen.

This event occurs frequently. Staff in crisis units are often inured to such threats and even to assaults themselves. Further history about the patient may help to speculate that the threat was a manifestation of the patient's fear, for example, of being committed. It is surprising to me that the resident did not comment to the patient on the threat at the time of the incident but turned and walked away. Threats are messages and require comment; to ignore them is to give a message that you do not care, that you are indifferent to suffering, or that you are disdainful. I would advise the clinician promptly to stop what he or she is doing and engage the patient in dialogue. My own strategy would be to say to the patient that I do not like being threatened and that it makes me angry and anxious. I comment that I imagine that the patient must be feeling the same way. Such a statement can be made in the midst of the busiest intervention. The main point is to convey to the patient that his or her threat has been heard and is being reacted to by the therapist. Occasionally, it is prudent to threaten the patient in return. Forensic specialists are frequently placed in positions where they must deal with threats. Tactics vary, but one response that I have heard is to tell the patient, in no uncertain terms, that the police will be called if the threat occurs again. I find such an approach quite appropriate if there exists no relationship with the patient; however, when an ongoing therapeutic relationship does exist, exploration of underlying dynamics is mandatory.

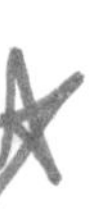

A final word should be said about telephone answering devices. The scenario for threats may be one of a long-term psychotherapy with a borderline or paranoid patient who is being treated by a therapist in solo private practice and who relies on a telephone answering machine. Answering machines are useful devices in some clinical situations, but they evoke anger in many people. For a patient struggling with intimacy and violent urges, the machine becomes symbolic of the therapist's neutral stance and may evoke rage. I would thus advise any therapist who is dealing with threats to deal with the patient directly and openly without the use of such a machine.

References

Bernstein H: Survey of threats and assaults directed toward therapists. Am J Psychother 35:542–549, 1981

Billowitz A, Pendleton L: Successful resolution of threats to a therapist. Hosp Community Psychiatry 39:782–783, 1988

Hoge SK, Gutheil TG: The prosecution of psychiatric patients for assaults on staff: a preliminary empirical study. Hosp Community Psychiatry 38:44–49, 1987

Lion JR: Training for battle: thoughts on managing aggressive patients. Hosp Community Psychiatry 38:882–884, 1987

Lion JR, Pasternak S: Countertransference reactions to violent patients. Am J Psychiatry 130:207–210, 1973

Lion JR, Reid W: Assaults Within Psychiatric Facilities. New York, Grune & Stratton, 1983

MacDonald J: A study of 100 homicidal patients. Am J Psychiatry 124:475–477, 1967

Chapter 6

Assaults With Weapons

William R. Dubin, M.D.

More than 40% of psychiatrists are assaulted at some time during their career (Bernstein 1981; Madden et al. 1976; Ruben et al. 1980; Tardiff and Maurice 1977; Whitman et al. 1976a). Of the many types of assaults, the most potentially dangerous is assault with a weapon. The definition of a weapon can vary—for example, knives or guns are indisputably weapons—but investigators often categorize any object that might be thrown as a weapon. The questions of intent further confounds the study of patient assaults. A patient may threaten a clinician with a gun or knife but have no intention of actually inflicting harm. Conversely, a patient may attack a psychiatrist with a chair, ashtray, or his or her hands and fully intend to cause serious injury or even death. These methodological issues complicate the study of armed assaults in clinical psychiatry.

There are anecdotal reports of clinicians being either threatened or harmed by an armed patient, but there is a paucity of information regarding such assaults. The purpose of this chapter is to review studies of assaults on psychiatrists by patients with weapons and to offer guidelines for managing such encounters.

A Review of the Literature

Studies of assaults against psychiatrists have found that many of the respondents were assaulted by patients with weapons. Hatti and col-

I thank Alicia Dubin and Marie Horn for their help with this manuscript and acknowledge Drs. Roy Whitman, Oran Dent, and Bea Armao who agreed to share their data with me.

leagues (1982) found that of 90 psychiatrists who had been assaulted, 25% had been attacked with fists, 23% with chairs, 4% with tables, 12% with ashtrays, 24% with guns, and 11% with knives. The assaults with guns or knives occurred exclusively in outpatient settings.

Bernstein (1981) noted that of the 60 assaults that were reported in his investigation, 72% consisted of hitting, biting, kicking, or choking. Eight assaults involved chairs, ashtrays, and a telephone; 2 involved a gun; 2 involved a knife; 1 involved an automobile; and 1 involved a set of crutches. Of therapists who received verbal threats, 20 were threatened by attack with feet or hands, 16 with a gun, 7 with a knife, and 7 with an office object.

Madden and colleagues (1976) reported that although the majority of assaults in their study involved a slap in the face or blow to the head, some psychiatrists reported having objects from their desk thrown at them. One psychiatrist in the study was shot by a patient.

In a follow-up of their initial study of assaults against psychiatrists, Dent and colleagues (O. B. Dent, R. M. Whitman, B. B. Armao, "Assault on the Therapist, Part II: The Attack, The Attacker, and The Attacked," unpublished manuscript, 1975) found that six therapists were threatened with a gun or knife, and six therapists were actually attacked with these weapons.

In a study of psychiatric residents, Ruben and colleagues (1980) found that weapons used by patients included purses, books, telephones, and ashtrays. Several attacks were made by hitting or pinching.

Gray (1989) found that of the 38 assaults against psychiatric residents, 1 involved a knife and 3 involved a thrown object. One assault was an attempted strangulation; the remainder of the assaults involved kicking, hitting, or other forms of physical contact.

The most detailed report of psychiatrists assaulted with weapons involved 32 psychiatrists; 17 were assaulted with a gun, and 15 were attacked by a patient with a knife (Dubin et al. 1988). These psychiatrists were part of a larger group of 91 psychiatrists who reported being assaulted in an outpatient setting during their career. The remaining 59 respondents experienced assaults by thrown objects or physical attacks. Of the psychiatrists who were assaulted with guns or knives, 67% were between the ages of 25 and 45, and 87% were male. Five psychiatrists were assaulted in their residency, 10 experienced the assault within the first 5 years out of their residency, and 4 respondents were assaulted 6–10 years following their psychiatric residency. The remaining 10 psychiatrists had been practicing from 11 to 20 years at the time of the assault. There was no relationship found between the level of experience and the seriousness of the assault. In other words, an experienced psychiatrist was just as likely to be assaulted with a gun or knife as was an inexperienced psychiatrist.

In this study, the mean duration of the assaults was 28.2 minutes with a gun and 5.4 minutes with a knife. Of the assaults with guns, nine occurred in private offices in office buildings; none occurred in community mental health centers. Similarly, of the 14 assaults with knives, 6 occurred in private offices in office buildings and only 1 occurred in a community mental health center setting.

Characteristics of the types of patients who committed assaults with a gun or knife can be summarized as follows: Of 31 patients, 24 were between the ages of 19 and 34; 23 were male; and 27 were white. Other demographic characteristics found that 23 had never been married, separated, or divorced. Almost half, 14 of the 31 patients, had not finished high school. There were two major diagnoses: 12 patients had personality disorder and 12 had schizophrenia. At the time of the assault, 12 patients were in psychotherapy and 13 were in combined drug therapy and psychotherapy. The predominant type of psychotherapy was insight oriented. Seven patients were on neuroleptics, and five were on antidepressants. The length of the sessions for the majority of the patients was 45–60 minutes. Nine patients were seen more than once a week, nine were treated once a week, and the remainder at variously longer intervals.

Of the patients who assaulted clinicians with a knife or gun, nine had been in treatment 1 month or less, seven patients had been in therapy up to 6 months, four had been in therapy up to 1 year, seven had been treated up to 5 years, and two patients had been in therapy more than 5 years. None of the assaults with guns resulted in significant harm to the psychiatrist or property damage. Similarly, of the 15 assaults with knives, none resulted in bodily harm, and only 2 resulted in property damage. Psychiatrists who were victims of assaults with fists or objects had significantly more bodily harm and property damage than psychiatrists who were only threatened with guns or knives. Precipitating events of armed assaults included limit setting, such as refusing to give a patient additional medication; psychodynamic issues, such as transference reactions; failure to set appropriate limits; and therapist error, such as the inappropriate handling of countertransference reactions.

The psychiatrists' emotional responses included fear of being hurt or killed, as well as anger. Fear was listed as the most frequent initial reaction to threats with guns and knives. Other common responses included attempts to remain calm and a desire to help. Psychiatrists who were assaulted with guns and knives tended to rely mainly on positive talking strategies such as speaking in a calming manner. Psychiatrists who responded with verbal or physical aggressiveness had a significantly higher percentage of injury or property damage.

Of the respondent psychiatrists in the study engaged in active treatment ($n = 81$), 48 (59%) continued to treat the patient after the assault. Five of the 12 psychiatrists who were injured also continued to treat their patients after the assault. It is significant to note that of the 48 psychiatrists who continued to treat their patients, 10 (21%) reported never discussing the incident with the patient and 16 (33%) reported making no changes in treatment modality, no changes in the treatment site, or taking no additional safety precautions!

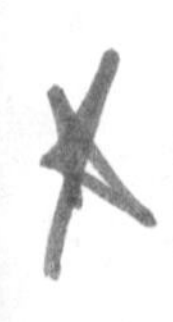

Indeed, only 20 (23%) of 87 respondents in this study reported having any security measures. Of the 87 psychiatrists, 31 (36%) reported having a moderate to strong feeling that the patient was potentially violent. Of the 20 psychiatrists with security precautions, 7 (35%) failed to implement them during the assault, and 52 of the attacked psychiatrists made no changes in their security precautions after the assault.

Physicians Killed by Patients

The incidence of physicians murdered by patients is unknown. Although there are anecdotes about such incidents, there is no database to help understand the circumstances surrounding homicides against a physician. The following are three reports that gave detailed accounts of psychiatrists who were shot by their patients.

Revitch

Revitch (1979) presented the case of a psychiatrist who was shot by a 53-year-old male patient he had been treating for depression for 13 years. On the day of the homicide, the patient sat calmly in the psychiatrist's waiting room for about 2 hours while the physician saw other patients. When the patient was called into the office and told that the visit would be short, the patient shot the doctor in the chest, killing him instantly.

During the 13 years of treatment, the patient had been hospitalized and given electroconvulsive therapy (ECT) on three occasions, the last hospitalization occurring 3–4 weeks prior to the homicide. After being discharged, the patient returned to work, where he was known as a very meticulous worker. Since the recent hospitalization, however, he had appeared to be somewhat depressed, as reflected by impairment in his work performance, attributed by the patient to the ECT treatment. Before the shooting, the patient had "brooded over his failure." Then, on the day of the incident, he resigned from his job despite objection from his employer and proceeded to the doctor's office, where he subsequently killed him. Later, when interviewed, the patient appeared to have no evidence of hallucinations, delusions, or paranoid thinking and stated he had no intention of killing the doctor but just wanted him to suffer "as I suffered."

Annis and Baker

Annis and Baker (1986) reported the death of a 38-year-old psychiatrist who was killed in an outpatient clinic of a state hospital. The 27-year-old patient who committed the homicide had a 5-year history of multiple commitments to the state hospital for threatening behavior secondary to persecutory delusions. Despite 10 hospitalizations, the patient showed little response to treatment and had been discharged at the request of his mother, who brought him in every few months for readmission. The slain psychiatrist was often the treating physician for this patient; they knew each other well.

The last hospital admission before the murder resembled previous ones. The patient was generally withdrawn, with little interaction except to relay his grandiose fantasies of being a prince from another planet. While in the hospital, there was an incident in which the patient knocked a female patient to the floor and began kicking her. When transferred to a closed ward, the patient stated that he would "run away, turn himself into a god of Mercury and get Dr. O.," the psychiatrist he ultimately killed. This verbalized hostility against the doctor was not new. The patient had threatened to kill the professional staff in general and his doctor in particular. The patient told Dr. O. that "he would collect other warrior gods from other planets and return to earth for a shoot-out, using shotguns, pistols, and other weapons." Approximately 1 month after the attack on the other patient, this assaultive patient was discharged from the hospital. Although remaining delusional, he was calm and cooperative. Six weeks after discharge, his psychotic symptoms worsened, and his aunt drove him to the hospital. He entered the reception area and opened his coat, exposing a double-barreled shotgun. He told the secretary that he wanted to see Dr. O. The secretary went to Dr. O.'s office and told him the patient "is out here with a shotgun. He says he wants to see you." Dr. O. rose from his desk and walked to the doorway, extending his hand in greeting. The patient opened fire, hitting Dr. O. in the chest, killing him instantly. After a "standoff" with the sheriff's deputies, the patient was finally captured and hospitalized. He was later found not guilty by reason of insanity.

Annis and Colleagues

In the third case study of a psychiatrist's murder, Annis and colleagues (1984) reviewed in detail the death of a 37-year-old psychiatrist who was killed by a 33-year-old former patient. When the patient was 10 years old, during a fit of anger, he had beaten his brother with a fire iron, causing cranial injuries with resultant mental retardation. Following this incident, the patient was hospitalized on a juvenile psychiatric ward 12 times during his adolescence. Eventually the patient went to college and obtained a master's degree in sociology. However, he was generally employed in menial jobs and was considered a loner. He was especially interested in guns, and he kept a collection of pistols and rifles. Once he severely injured his right arm after dropping a loaded Colt .45 revolver.

The patient next came to psychiatric attention in 1981 when he was involved in a high-speed chase (in excess of 100 miles an hour). He underwent psychiatric evaluation and was subsequently committed to a secure forensic unit at the state hospital after being found incompetent to stand trial. The patient was started on antipsychotic medications. He became cooperative and reasonable. However, he was eccentric with paranoid ideas but manifested no gross hallucinations or delusional thinking. He was transferred from the forensic unit to the state hospital, and, after 5 months, he appeared to be well behaved and not psychotic. He was subsequently discharged to a group home. He was described in the group home as superficial and brief, but polite. He rarely missed any of his three, daily 10-mg doses of haloperidol. While in the group home, the patient had a part-time job in the patient library at a nearby hospital. Approximately 2 months after discharge from the state hospital, the patient attempted to purchase a .38 caliber pistol using an expired revoked driver's license as proof of his identity. After the 3-day waiting period, the patient purchased the gun. He resigned from his job at the hospital. Around this time, it was noted by the staff that the patient was more untidy, and his personal appearance began to decline. He stopped bathing. He became unkempt in his dressing, his hair went unbrushed, and he began to miss medications.

It was noted that on the morning of the murder the patient was unusually cheerful. He was late and unable to make his scheduled appointment with his regular psychiatrist. He was told, however, that if he would wait he would be seen by Dr. W. After a period of time, Dr. W. walked into the lobby and asked to see another patient. Dr. W. and the patient left together and went to his office. Minutes later the patient left the lobby unnoticed and walked down the same passage. When he came to Dr. W.'s door, he pushed the door open and stepped into the room, stating in a calm voice, "Are you a psychiatrist?" Dr. W. answered, "Yes, I am." The patient then said, "Then I've got something for you." He drew the pistol and fired in Dr. W.'s direction until the gun was empty. The patient then stated, "I cannot believe I did that." He slowly walked out of the hospital as if nothing had happened. He was subsequently arrested, found guilty of first-degree murder, and sentenced to life imprisonment without parole.

These three reported cases graphically depict the tragic deaths of three psychiatrists.

Management of the Armed Patient

Confrontation with an armed patient may be the endpoint of a deteriorating clinical situation. The clinician often fails to intervene because his or her psychological defenses tend to minimize or disregard the threat. The clinician may also be unable to set appropriate limits. Additionally, rarely does a psychiatrist give preparatory thought to the physical layout of the office or develop a security plan.

The most effective intervention with an armed patient is anticipation of the risks of violence for a given patient, recognizing one's own blind spots in assessing these risks. A psychiatrist should also work in an office that minimizes the risk of an overt assault.

Psychological Defenses

A major impediment to effective intervention with a violent patient is the psychological defense of denial. Denial helps clinicians cope with unbearable anxiety and feelings of helplessness and is manifested by the failure to gather unflattering or anxiety-producing data from a threatening or intimidating patient (Lion and Pasternak 1973). Madden and colleagues (1976) found that 55% of psychiatrists felt retrospectively that they could have anticipated an assault. Similarly, Dubin and colleagues (1988) found that 36% of psychiatrists had moderate to strong feelings that their patient was potentially assaultive. Despite their clinical intuition, however, the psychiatrists in these studies did not pursue those clinical issues that might attenuate the risk of assault.

Patients should routinely be asked about ownership of weapons, ammunition, previous use of weapons, lethal skills (e.g., training in martial arts), past criminal acts, past violent acts, and a history of driving offenses. If the patient owns a weapon, the patient's fantasies and intentions regarding the weapon must be discussed. In addition to the patient interview, information may be obtained from family members, prior clinical records, other clinical evaluations, and, when appropriate, police arrest records. Tardiff (1989) provided a useful clinical profile that, analogous to suicide risk factors, outlines risk factors for predicting short-term violence (days to a week). These factors include the following:

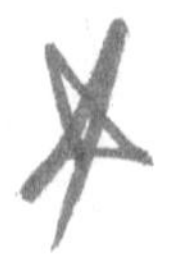

1. Appearance of the patient: signs of alcohol or drug use, agitation, anger, degree of compliance with procedures, or disorganized behavior
2. Degree of detail or plan of a threat of violence
3. Available means of inflicting serious injury (e.g., purchase or possession of a gun)
4. History of violence or other impulsive behaviors, including suicide, destruction of property, reckless driving, reckless spending, sexual acting out, or other antisocial behaviors

5. Target(s) of past violence toward others
6. Degree of injury in violence toward others
7. Circumstances and patterns of escalation of violence toward others
8. History of physical abuse as a child or occurrence of other familial violence as a child
9. Presence of alcohol or drug use, particularly cocaine, amphetamines, anxiolytics, sedatives, and hallucinogens
10. Presence of other organic disorders including, and other medical disorders affecting, the central nervous system
11. Presence of any psychotic psychopathology, particularly paranoid delusions or command hallucinations
12. Presence of organic, borderline, or antisocial personality disorder
13. Being in a demographic group with increased prevalence of violence: young male, lower socioeconomic groups

Setting Limits

A striking finding when violent episodes are reviewed is the failure of the psychiatrist to set limits for patients who lack adequate internal controls (Dubin et al. 1988). There are certain patients who are unable to control or limit their behavior, and psychiatrists must actively impose external controls. Insight, empathy, and understanding are not enough to deter violence. Any threat or any behavior that is inappropriately aggressive should be dealt with immediately. Often the fear of damaging the therapeutic alliance leads psychiatrists to minimize a patient's actions. In the most extreme example of this mistaken notion reported by Dubin and colleagues, 21% of psychiatrists who continued to see their patients after being threatened with a weapon never discussed the incident with the patient.

An example of a failure to set limits is demonstrated in a vignette in which a psychiatrist was threatened by a patient with a knife (Dubin et al. 1988). The same patient in an earlier session had thrown an ashtray at the psychiatrist. The therapist never said to the patient that such behavior was dangerous and unacceptable. He felt that he could overpower the patient, a small woman, and therefore never thought it necessary to discuss the incident.

Another example of failure to set limits is a case in which a psychiatrist had treated a patient for 8 years. During this time, the patient constantly made threats that he would "cut up" the psychiatrist. At no time did the psychiatrist state that such threats were unacceptable. During the eighth year of treatment, the psychiatrist's pregnant wife started working as the office receptionist. When the patient stated that he was going to "cut her up," the psychiatrist panicked over the threat and immediately wanted to transfer the patient to another therapist. The entire episode might have been averted if limit setting had occurred 7 years earlier.

In an excellent book on limit setting, Green and colleagues (1988) concluded that effective limit setting involves a clear identification of the specific maladaptive behaviors that need to be altered. They also noted that precise articulation of the consequences that will follow if inappropriate behaviors persist is equally important. The authors stressed that the therapist should periodically reaffirm the limits by reminding the patient of the specific behavior that has been targeted for specific consequences. They further observed that if the therapist lacks clarity in his or her thinking or communications to the patient concerning inappropriate behaviors, the intervention may, instead, confuse and disorganize the patient. Whenever feasible, confrontational and interpretative intervention should precede the imposition of limits because these maneuvers afford the patients greater flexibility in exercising their own autonomy and discretion. When appropriate, it is important to engage the patient in decision making as to the types of limits set. The basic philosophy of limit setting is to contain and counteract maladaptive behaviors that interfere with psychotherapy and threaten its viability or the safety of the patient and/or therapist (Green et al. 1988). The clinician must first identify such behaviors to the patient. The final step is to specify the consequences that will ensue should the patient ignore the explicitly detailed limits. Consequences may include alteration of the treatment setting, a change in therapist, or termination of treatment.

Thackery (1987) stated that limit setting should never be presented as a request, advice, bribe, punishment, or challenge. Instead, a patient should be offered alternatives. He defined indirect limit setting in which a patient is given a choice of several acceptable alternatives. The offer of several alternatives divides the patient's will to resist, and generally the patient will choose the most acceptable alternative. Thus, the clinician maintains control by limiting choices while giving the patient responsibility for choosing.

Management of Threats

The management of threats is an important element in lowering the risk of assaults with weapons. Denial may lead a clinician to minimize or ignore a threat. However, *all* threats must be taken with an equal degree of seriousness. A threat, regardless of how insignificant it may appear, should be examined. If the psychiatrist feels the threat is serious, and there is a possibility that the patient will act on the threat, other colleagues, or if appropriate the police, should be notified. If the police fail to act or provide help, the district attorney's office should be notified. Because a district attorney is concerned about the political ramifications of a potentially catastrophic event, this contact may be more helpful. If the threats persist, it is crucial to let the patient know that the psychiatrist has notified authorities and colleagues and that the threat has been publicized. Too often there is a tendency not to discuss the threats, and it is only following some catastrophic event that it becomes known that the psychiatrist was threatened.

Billowitz and Pendleton (1988) discussed a protocol, summarized below, that was successful in resolving a prototypic threat to a therapist.

> A 32-year-old female clinical psychologist received a threatening letter from a patient, stating that if the therapist did not acquiesce to bizarre and regressive sexual acts, there would be escalating consequences of an unspecified nature. The management of the threat focused on three areas: therapist safety, lines of communication, and sources of other information and guidance.
>
> Plans were made for situations in which the therapist might confront the patient (e.g., in the hospital, the parking lot, or the home). Hospital security accompanied the therapist to her home, and clerical personnel were cautioned and reminded not to give out home telephone numbers. The hospital security director, chief executive officer, and attorney were promptly notified and consulted. The patient's former therapist was also notified. Throughout this entire notification process, the hospital's attorney was the only individual to whom the identity of the patient was disclosed. Several psychiatrists in the community and attorneys were informally consulted, as was the chief county prosecutor.
>
> Finally, a letter was sent to the patient by the program director. The letter stated, "Your letter to Dr. A. was received earlier this week and has been reviewed by the authorities in the hospital legal office and administration as well as by psychiatrists. All agreed that your letter

contains abnormal thinking and demonstrates a need for psychiatric help. Most importantly, we further agree that your letter contains harassment and threats that cannot be tolerated. Should any further letters be sent by you they will not be opened by Dr. A. or myself. Instead such letters will be forwarded directly through the hospital to the proper legal authorities for immediate legal action" (Billowitz and Pendleton 1988, pp. 782–783).

Four days later, a letter of apology arrived from the patient, explaining his behavior and containing a plea for help. The patient was referred to another therapist in a different hospital. Four years after the incident, the patient had made no further contact with the therapist.

This case illustrates a well-thought-out, well-planned intervention. The issues of therapist safety, lines of communication, and other sources of information for guidance are criteria that can be applied to most threats.

Treatment Settings

The choice of treatment setting can also be a factor that encourages or discourages violence. Patients who have histories of violence, or who are psychotic and have tenuous impulse control, should not be seen in private homes or commercial office settings. Hospital settings, emergency departments, crisis centers, or medical centers where there are sufficient personnel to help control a patient are safer. Richmond and Ruparel (1980) suggested that for patients with the potential for violence, multiple caregiving using a clinic's staff resources may be a preferable treatment alternative. A clinician is always available, and staff are present to help set limits and physically control the patient when necessary. In addition, the transference and countertransference feelings are diluted as the patient has contact with a variety of therapists.

Office Safety

In dealing with aggressive patients, the most effective intervention is prevention. The clinician must plan for the possibility of being threatened or assaulted. This includes evaluating one's office and work area to ensure a safe physical environment. Tardiff (1989) suggested that clinicians should use solid furniture, including heavy chairs, or "beanbag" chairs, which are difficult to move or throw. Ashtrays and heavy objects should not be used in the office; pillows and other soft objects on chairs may be useful as shields. Clinicians should have either panic buttons or prearranged signals to the outside community so that a colleague or receptionist may be alerted of danger. The receptionist should have a panic button or a signal to warn the psychiatrist if a threatening patient or situation is developing in the reception area.

When interviewing patients who have been violent or who are potentially explosive, clinicians should pay attention to their own attire (Tardiff 1989). Eyeglasses, necklaces, and earrings should be removed. Ties should be taken off or tucked into a shirt.

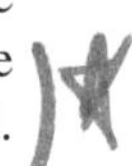

The Armed Patient: Intervention

Because of the paucity of studies of encounters with armed patients, there are few guidelines to assist the clinician. As with all violence, however, there are certain principles essential to achieving a successful resolution of a confrontation with an armed patient. Recognition of the dynamics of violence is critical to any intervention. Violence is a defense against passivity and helplessness and represents an effort to protect the patient from loss of self-esteem. Therefore, verbal or physical aggression by the clinician is likely to shift the dynamic toward violence. Ruben and colleagues (1980) found that psychiatric residents who were highly irritable and said that they would become aggressive if confronted with a violent patient were significantly more likely to be assaulted during their residency. In contrast, verbal interventions, coupled with an initial response of fear and a desire to help, generally resulted in the most successful outcome (Dubin et al. 1988). Verbal or physical aggression leads to increased personal injury and property destruction.

Whitman and colleagues (1976b) described the coping techniques of therapists who were threatened or assaulted by patients. The authors categorized therapist responses into coping mechanisms with a variety of responses.

Interruption was a technique in which therapists removed themselves or the patient either briefly or for longer periods of time from the ongoing interchange. For example, a therapist might excuse himself or herself to make a telephone call to speak with a colleague, or leave the room for a prearranged commitment. At other times, a therapist might ask a patient to compose himself or herself in the waiting room or to return in a day or a week for another appointment.

A second type of coping technique was physical restraint in which the clinician sought help from other such psychiatric aides, police, or security guards. Most of the physical restraint techniques occurred in inpatient settings.

A third technique—minimization of self as a threat—included remaining still, shaking hands, opening the door, sitting (rather than standing), presenting a calm demeanor, showing interest by leaning forward, interviewing in daytime, and letting the patient sit closest to the door. This response could be characterized as attempting to make the therapist appear physically smaller.

The most important technique, according to the authors, was verbal coping techniques. The verbal responses used by therapists showed variety and ingenuity. Table 6–1 demonstrates the wide range of verbal coping techniques used (Whitman et al. 1976b).

Other interventions included fighting back, fleeing, anticipating the danger by responding to nonverbal cues during the interview, removing potential weapons from sight, having the patient sit down, ringing an alarm, or making other noise. Several of the respondents in this study dealt with the patient's threat of aggression by encouraging physical displacement of anger to objects or by allowing the patient to take a walk.

Respondents also described countertransference maneuvers in which they thought of the patient as someone in need, as hopeless, and therefore weak. By using this technique, the therapist was able to decrease his or her own anxiety.

Tardiff (1989) suggested that if a patient appears in a treatment setting with a weapon, such as a gun, there should be exposure to as few staff as possible. For example, if a psychiatrist is aware of such a patient in the reception area, there should be an immediate retreat to the office, and the patient should not be engaged in the reception area. Tardiff suggested that if trapped, the clinician should acknowledge the patient with a neutral and obvious remark (e.g., "I see you have a gun"). The therapist should appear calm and not be intimidating, confrontational, or argumentative. The clinician should encourage the patient to talk during the initial phases of confrontation and explore the patient's concerns. There should be no attempt to take the weapon from the

patient. If the patient is willing to surrender the weapon, it should be put on a desk or on the floor. The clinician should never reach for the gun or tell the patient to drop the gun. This could result in its discharge.

A clinician who is threatened by a patient with a gun should recognize that the firearm is almost invariably an expression of feelings of inadequacy and fear. Therefore, Thackery (1987) recommended that the clinician attempt to speak directly to the underlying psychological issue. If a short time passes without the patient's actually firing the gun, the likelihood of its eventual use is diminished. Initially, however, the clinician should comply with whatever demand the patient may make and take special care to avoid upsetting the patient further. The clinician must not attempt to talk the patient into surrendering the firearm but rather suggest that the patient point the weapon away while they talk. At an appropriate time, the clinician may suggest that the patient place the weapon in a safe, neutral place.

Bowie (1989) stated that interactions with assaultive patients should be done in a calm, easy style as if speaking to a friend or peer. Suggestions for approaching assaultive patients include letting the patients know that their position is clearly understood and attempting to engage the patients in topics that will motivate their self-interest. It is important to identify areas in which the patient's viewpoint is correct rather than initially trying to demonstrate the areas in which the patient's viewpoint is wrong. The alliance will be enhanced if the clinician can identify similarities between himself or herself and the patient. Bowie underscored the critical point that fighting is a last resort, when no other option is available, and must be done to save a life or to avoid a major injury. Clinicians should not engage in physical aggression when other options are available, when persuasion can deter the patient, when the patient has a weapon that he or she will use, or when help is coming and the patient can be stalled or diverted.

In discussing the strategy of fleeing from a threatening patient, Bowie (1989) underscored several important issues. He suggested that the clinician leave when a situation seems totally uncontrollable. Before leaving, the therapist should consider what must be done to escape and the nearest safe place. When leaving, the clinician should not run as in a panic reaction but should leave as a positive action. The clinician should run toward a place of safety and not just away from danger. Once beginning the escape, the clinician should not hesitate or stop until free and clear.

Table 6–1. Examples of verbal coping techniques

Technique	Example
1. Ask for words versus acting.	1. Why don't you tell me how angry you feel rather than swinging at me?
2. Permit ventilation of anger.	2.
a) Encourage specificity.	a) Why don't you tell me exactly what you are angry with me about?
b) With explicit approval.	b) I can take your anger.
3. Casual talk.	3. Did you see the game last night?
4. Emphasize purpose of interchange; clarify role.	4. I am here to understand you rather than to be your punching bag.
5. Interpretation.	5.
a) Transference.	a) I think you are really angry with your father.
b) Make a diagnosis and anticipate danger.	b) You are having an anxiety reaction and you often attack people when you feel this way.
c) As a manifestation of frustration.	c) You want to kill me because you are very agitated.
d) As temporary.	d) You feel like killing me right now, but I feel that you will get over it.
e) Point out generalization.	e) You want to kill anybody that gets in your way.
f) Identify displacement.	f) It's your boss you are really angry at.
g) Motivational questioning.	g) Where do you think these murderous feelings are coming from?
6. Be honest with patient.	6. I realize now that I must have hurt your feelings.
7. Be sympathetically firm.	7. I really can't let you hit me.

Technique	Example
8. Get patient's agreement to rules of therapy.	8. Let's agree that any physical blows are out of order here.
9. Exhortative measures or commands; shouting.	9. Now stop this immediately! Put that gun down!
10. Anticipate negative consequences in future. a) Legal retaliation. b) No headlines or fame.	10. a) If you kill me, you will go to the electric chair. b) Your picture won't be in the paper if you shoot me.
11. Assurance of not hurting the patient.	11. I am not going to do anything to harm you.
12. Threaten with immediate incarceration.	12. I'll call the guard if you strike me.
13. Label in another dimension.	13. You'll feel different after a good night's sleep.
14. Humor.	14. Tell me exactly what's going through your mind (as the patient holds a gun on the therapist).
15. Talk about a significant reality issue.	15. Let's talk about your medication.
16. List of things to take care of.	16. You need to talk to your employer, the Veterans Administration contact representative, and the rehabilitation counselor this coming week.
17. Have patient's interest at heart.	17. You know that I have already sent your forms to the insurance company.
18. Stop uncovering questions.	18. Let's not talk any more about Vietnam.
19. Comment on how therapist was made to feel.	19. You are frightening me.

continued

Table 6–1. Examples of verbal coping techniques *(continued)*

Technique	Example
20. Shame.	20. You are behaving like a child who isn't getting his or her way.
21. Let the patient know he or she can leave if he or she wants to.	21. Maybe you would rather leave than lose control of yourself.
22. Empathize. a) With the patient's current dilemma. b) With motivational dilemma.	22. a) You feel so angry that you would like to hit me. b) If that happened to me, I'd feel like doing that, too.
23. Counterexpression of hostility.	23. I'm angry, too, but it won't get us anyplace.
24. Appeal to a superordinate principle.	24. Guns are not allowed in the Veterans Administration hospital.

Source. Adapted from Whitman et al. 1976b.

Conclusion

Management of violent patients is a major challenge to clinicians. Intervention with violent and armed patients represents the ultimate threat to clinicians. The very thought of confronting an armed patient is so anxiety provoking that most clinicians suppress this notion altogether. However, there are steps that clinicians can take to reduce the risk of assaults and injury.

Psychiatrists must routinely and thoroughly explore the patient's past history regarding previous episodes of violence, ownership of weapons and ammunition, and associated fantasies. Threats should be explored in detail and treated seriously. The factors outlined by Tardiff (1989) for assessing violence should be a routine part of every evaluation. Psychiatrists must become more adept at setting limits and be aware of their own denial, which can circumvent this important process.

Treatment offices should be made as environmentally safe as possible. Physicians should develop security plans and rehearse them periodically. Psychiatrists who have any doubts about management of aggressive or threatening patients should immediately seek consultation with a colleague. The threat of violence with a weapon is a terrifying experience. However, by implementing the above strategies, the risk of harm can be reduced.

References

Annis LV, Baker CA: A psychiatrist's murder in a mental hospital. Hosp Community Psychiatry 38:505–506, 1986

Annis LV, McClaren HA, Baker CA: Who kills us: case study of a clinician's murder, in Violence in the Medical Care Setting: A Survival Guide. Edited by Turner JT. Rockville, MD, Aspen, 1984, pp 19–31

Bernstein HA: Survey of threats and assaults directed toward psychotherapists. Am J Psychother 35:542–549, 1981

Billowitz A, Pendleton L: Successful resolution of threats to a therapist. Hosp Community Psychiatry 39:782–783, 1988

Bowie V: Coping With Violence. Sydney, Australia, Karibuni Press, 1989

Dubin WR, Wilson SJ, Mercer C: Assaults against psychiatrists in outpatient settings. J Clin Psychiatry 49:338–345, 1988

Gray GE: Assaults by patients against residents at a public psychiatric hospital. Academic Psychiatry 13:81–86, 1989

Green SA, Goldberg RL, Goldstein DM, et al: Limit Setting in Clinical Practice. Washington, DC, American Psychiatric Press, 1988

Hatti S, Dubin WR, Weiss KJ: A study of circumstances surrounding patient assaults on psychiatrists. Hosp Community Psychiatry 33:660–661, 1982

Lion JR, Pasternak SA: Countertransference reaction to violent patients. Am J Psychiatry 130:207–209, 1973

Madden DJ, Lion JR, Penna MW: Assaults on psychiatrists by patients. Am J Psychiatry 133:422–425, 1976

Revitch E: Patients who kill their physician. The Journal of the Medical Society of New Jersey 76:429–431, 1979

Richmond JS, Ruparel MK: Management of violent patients in a psychiatric walk-in clinic. J Clin Psychiatry 41:370–373, 1980

Ruben I, Walkon G, Yamamoto J: Physical attacks on psychiatric residents by patients. J Nerv Ment Dis 168:243–245, 1980

Tardiff K: Assessment and Management of Violent Patients. Washington, DC, American Psychiatric Press, 1989

Tardiff K, Maurice WL: The care of violent patients by psychiatrists: a tale of two cities. Canadian Psychiatry Association Journal 22:83–86, 1977

Thackery M: Therapeutics for Aggression. New York, Human Sciences Press, 1987

Whitman, RM, Armao BB, Dent OB: Assaults on the therapist. Am J Psychiatry 133:426–431, 1976a

Whitman RM, Armao BB, Dent OB: Assaults on the therapist, III: coping and disposition. Paper presented at the 129th annual meeting of the American Psychiatric Association, Miami, Florida, May 13, 1976b

Chapter 7

Managing Countertransference Reactions to Aggressive Patients

Gary J. Maier, M.D., and Gregory J. Van Rybroek, Ph.D., J.D.

In nearly all states the standards that govern civil commitment have been narrowed to mental illness and dangerousness. As a result, psychiatric hospitals now house a subset of patients: the irritable, angry, and aggressive patient (Maier and Van Rybroek 1990). Managing aggressive behavior, however, is still in the "shadow" of psychiatry for a number of reasons, including underdeveloped clinical theory, uncoordinated training, and poor management of staff countertransference reactions (Lion 1987). Because aggressive events are threatening and cause injury, the normal reactions of fear and anger have also hindered rational progress in making the work environment safe. The very techniques required to manage aggression—seclusion, physical restraint, ambulatory restraint, and chemical restraint—activate unpleasant feelings because they strike at the basic values of freedom and dignity. When seclusion becomes the principal way to manage the acutely aggressive patient, it is easy to conclude that out of sight (seclusion) is out of mind (denial). Denying that a significant number of our patients are aggressive is the primary factor impeding progress in the management and treatment of these patients.

Administrators and clinicians need to become more aware that assault is an occupational hazard of working with aggressive inpatients. To improve the quality of the workplace, we need to break through the traditional denial that has shrouded this issue. Clinical theory that accurately outlines the sequence of events that occur in a single aggressive episode must be developed. The dynamics that drive repetitive aggression, called "aggression cycles," and a description of the basic nodal points found embedded in them need clarification. Being aware that aggression can cause strong reactions in the staff working with the aggressive patient, and that these reactions can have a lasting impact that will affect the ability of the staff to continue to provide humane care to such patients, is essential. The development of a countertransference policy is an important way that administrators and clinicians can demonstrate that they are aware of the problem and that they support efforts to care for the caregivers.

In this chapter, we describe a clinical model of aggression as a phased process with a discernible structure. Understanding the phases is valuable in understanding when and how to intervene to prevent aggression or to bring it to safe resolution. The model suggests the need for aggression postmortems and for process meetings (called Me-Time). We conclude by describing how staff develop countertransference reactions to these patients and suggest a way to identify and resolve these reactions.

Understanding Aggression

Clinical observation of patient-patient aggression demonstrates that the elements of each aggressive event follow a similar course. Further observation allows us to conclude that although the course of single aggressive events is similar, the course of events that occurs when there are repeated episodes of aggression has unique phases. From these observations a comprehensive clinical model was developed for understanding and managing aggression (Maier et al. 1987, 1988; Van Rybroek and Maier 1987). The model consists of two dynamic processes: the process that occurs during a single aggressive event, called the linear aggression sequence, and the more complicated process that results when aggression becomes repetitive, called the physical aggression cycle.

Linear Aggression Sequence

Aggression occurring in a medical setting can be regarded as a linear process that may be broken down into six phases: 1) "preaggression," 2) aggression, 3) control, 4) diagnosis and assessment, 5) treatment and management, and 6) aggression postmortem (Figure 7–1).

Because the first three phases of the aggression sequence can flow into each other in a rapid fashion and may cause physiological arousal

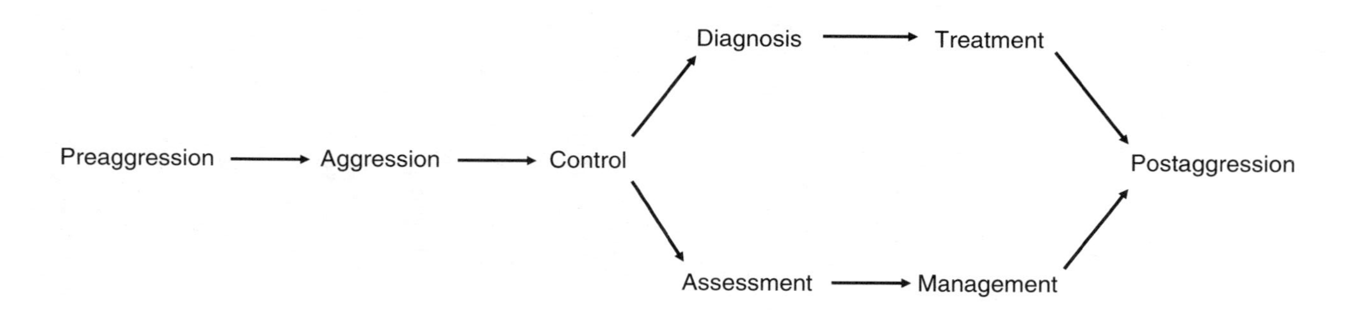

Figure 7–1. The linear aggression sequence. The linear aggression sequence in an inpatient setting consists of six phases. In medical settings, the difference between the two tracts of the latter phases is often a source of confusion. A number of disciplines—security guards, prison guards, police, SWAT members, and military teams—are charged with the responsibility of controlling and managing aggressive persons. Staff who work in medical settings share this responsibility and use similar interventions. They are also able to diagnose and treat these patients, and, to the degree that aggressive behavior is part of the illness, treatment reduces aggression. The postaggression phase recognizes the need to document and even research each aggressive event, unfettered by incipient countertransference feelings, which often contaminate fact finding that can lead to better management and treatment techniques.

in the staff, they have been difficult to separate. Further, these phases are at times poorly differentiated, so staff reactions to them can become confused, and interventions can become misplaced. Phases four and five are bimodal; two separate but related functions occur during each phase. The following description of the characteristics and boundaries of each phase outlines the general structure of these processes. Because the processes can be complex, this outline is an approximation of the phases themselves.

Preaggression phase. Monahan (1981) identified the complex relationship that exists among the various factors that determine the emergence of aggressive behavior. The origins of this phase can be directly related to the theoretical orientation of the clinician. For example, for a Freudian, the preaggressive phase may begin as early as the emergence of dental aggression in infancy (Perls 1947). At the other end of the spectrum, a behaviorist may limit the origins of the phase to the various contingencies in operation moments before the aggression erupted. Although Tanke and Yesavage (1985) demonstrated that the Brief Psychiatric Rating Scale can be used to identify patients who will aggress but who do not give verbal cues prior to their aggression, research of this type has not yet resulted in the development of reliable etiological typologies. Nevertheless, Harris and Varney (1983) reported that patient-patient aggression is usually the product of a direct interaction between patients. Patients report a number of reasons they aggress against each other. These range from a simple "payback" for a previous transgression to the "acting out" of a command hallucination. Whatever the origins, the preaggression phase typically ends with either a verbal (gestural) threat or a physically aggressive act.

Aggression phase. The aggression phase begins with a verbal threat or an act of physical aggression (Dubin 1985). This phase may consist of punches, kicks, bites, and scratches. Often one patient is the manifest aggressor and another patient (or a staff member) is the manifest victim. The phase continues until the aggressor regains self-control or the staff intervenes and subdues the patient. When staff members witness the onset of this phase, they must intervene, either by talking down or by taking down the aggressive patient. This phase involves engaging the patient until the staff has established control. This phase can be as short as the time it takes a patient to make a verbal threat or as long as it takes a SWAT team to gain control over an aggressive patient who has taken a hostage (Mendota Mental Health Institute 1989b).

Control phase. During the control phase, the aggressive behavior is stopped, either because the patient develops self-control or because of the staff intervenes. In situations where staff arrive after the patient has stopped the aggressive act, the control phase is synonymous with the development of self-control by the patient and the patient's resulting ability to demonstrate responsibility. In other situations, staff must actively intervene to stop the aggression; that often means they must physically control the patient (Thackery 1987). In these situations, control is initiated and maintained through physical or chemical restraint or both and, as appropriate, seclusion. When the patient has finally regained self-control, the staff may impose a probationary period during which the patient must demonstrate that staff directions can and will be accepted. This period often occurs while the patient is secluded. The control phase ends when the staff gives the patient the responsibility for self-control in an open environment.

The act of aggression breaks the trust that is the bond of the therapeutic alliance. One cannot provide therapy to a person who is attacking. Consequently, staff members become empowered to utilize "police" powers during the control phase. At the same time, the patient loses certain rights. It is for this obvious reason that it is important to distinguish between the concepts of control and management that are not based on trust, and treatment or therapy that is indeed based on trust. This fundamental difference is often not sufficiently understood by administrators, training directors, or patient advocates.

Diagnosis and assessment. There is a difference between *diagnosis* and *assessment.* Using the medical model (Lion 1972), the term *diagnosis* is reserved for the process of determining the presence of medical or psychiatric illness. Unfortunately, medical or psychiatric diagnoses are often of little value in determining the probability of future aggression because aggressive behavior is seldom pathognomonic of any specific disorder, and, worse, aggression can be associated with nearly any medical or psychiatric disorder. Diagnosis follows the traditional medical and psychiatric process and is based on history, physical examination, laboratory tests, the patient's mental status, neurological examination, psychological tests, and other special medical procedures such as computed tomography scan, X ray, or electroencephalogram. The process can take from a few days to several weeks and may include clinical trials on medication. Currently diagnoses are made in the DSM-IV (American Psychiatric Association 1994) format.

The term *assessment* is reserved for the process of determining the probability that a patient will become aggressive in the immediate future (hours, days, or weeks) (Tardiff 1989). Assessment for aggression potential is done by a review of the patient's history of aggressive behavior at home, at school, at work, and, if applicable, in hospitals, in correctional facilities, or in the armed services. The relationship between the aggressive behavior and environmental and situational factors is important. The description of aggressive behaviors outlined in the Overt Aggression Scale by Yudofsky and colleagues (1986)—including aggression against others, aggression against property, threats toward others, and aggression against self—is useful in establishing meaningful clinical categories. These categories can be used to look for patterns that may then help determine the long-term management plan. Although past behavior is still the most reliable predictor of future behavior, patients who manifest behavior from more than one category are often more dangerous than those who act out with only one pattern (Depp 1976; Silver and Yudofsky 1987).

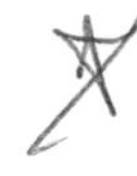

Treatment and management phase. The term *treatment* is used in the classic medical sense. Thus, *treatment* refers to all the traditional approaches used to help mentally ill persons and includes psychotherapy, psychopharmacology, and some behavioral approaches based on learning theory. When aggressive behaviors are closely associated with the psychiatric illness (e.g., paranoid schizophrenia), treating the illness will often significantly reduce the aggression. In this construct, the aggressive behavior is considered to be a sign of illness because the treatment does, or appears to, correct the primary pathology. Frequently, however, the aggressive behavior is characterological, learned, or only coincidentally associated with the psychiatric condition. In these cases, the terms *manage* and *management* are used to refer to the interventions. These terms refer to approaches used to exert external control over aggressive behavior. Talk-down and take-down procedures, seclusion, and ambulatory restraints are good examples. Clinicians may need to continue specific treatment or management techniques to help a patient maintain behavioral control for short periods of time or for the indefinite future.

Aggression postmortems. Following each aggressive episode of any significance, an independent fact finder should review all aspects of the aggressive event and then meet with the principals involved to understand from their perspectives what happened, what might have prevented it, and, once started, what would have brought the event under control more quickly and with less trauma. Utilizing this procedure allows each aggressive event to become a learning event and not just a traumatic event. A report that describes the incident and the outcomes and makes recommendations to senior clinicians and administrators should follow. Careful review of the data over time may suggest new ways to intervene and can also identify patterns of aggression unique to the specific unit or facility that can suggest alternative ways of responding.

Physical Aggression Cycle

The second component of this model consists of identifying the processes that occur when aggression becomes repetitive. Although several authors (Kaplan and Wheeler 1980; McGee 1985; Rada 1981) have described cyclical patterns of aggression, these patterns have not been incorporated into a general model, nor have the authors focused on the critical role that staff countertransference plays in maintaining the cyclical process. The following describes these processes from the perspective of the staff, with specific reference to the need to identify and resolve staff feelings. The description of the physical aggression cycle from the patient's perspective is described in our comprehensive model (Maier et al. 1988) and elsewhere (Binder 1979; Binder and McCoy 1983).

Description of the cycle. Physical aggression often results in the chain of events illustrated in Figure 7–2. The first three phases of the process are the same as in the linear process. Staff respond rapidly to the patient-aggressor. They secure the patient by talk down or take down and, if necessary, use seclusion to control the patient.

After the patient is controlled, staff will spontaneously inquire

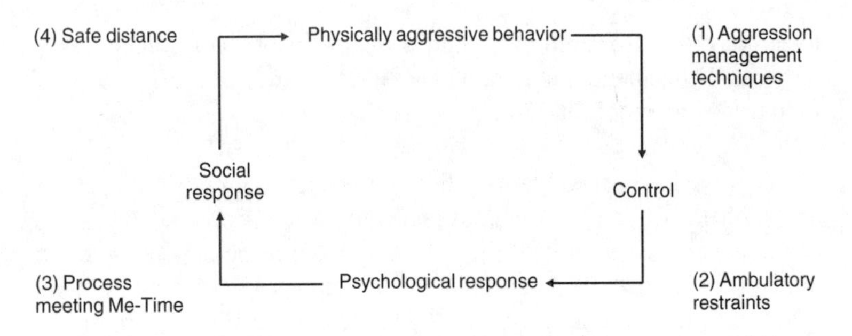

Figure 7–2. The physical aggression cycle: clinical perspective. The cardinal points of the cycle—physically aggressive behavior, control, psychological response, and social response—present the normal progression of clinician-patient dynamics that can result from an aggressive episode. The midpoints 1–4 represent the points where patients and staff can make the most effective interventions.

about possible physical injuries. They will not ask whether coworkers were frightened by the aggression or were angry that the patient put them in such jeopardy. If they recognize that they have these feelings themselves, they wait until after work to share them. Because the usual process of dealing with aggression in the work setting does not include discussion about staff feelings of fear, anger, rage, or a sense of helplessness, these feelings may go undetected and unresolved (Adler 1972; Cornfield and Fielding 1980; Kaplan and Wheeler 1983; Lion and Pasternak 1980; Madden and Lion 1976). The feelings, however, will not go away.

The secluded patient is usually released before the staff has time to process what conscious feelings they can identify. Staff and other patients may prepare for the patient's return with unresolved feelings. It is the accumulation of denied feeling that contributes to the creation of a cyclical process. Unresolved staff countertransference feelings[1] take over the process. As a result, when the patient is released from

[1] *Countertransference reactions* in this chapter refers to any staff feelings, conscious or unconscious, derived from the patient-staff relationship. In this chapter, we deal only with the fear, anger, hate, and rage spectrum of feelings because they are specifically aroused by aggression.

seclusion, some staff (and some patients) will remain physically and emotionally distant, thereby minimizing therapeutic contact. The distrust and anger the staff and other patients feel may be evident to the patient and cause the patient to feel alienated. Given this response, it is probable that a small incident will evoke another act of aggression and begin the cycle again (Alaron et al. 1988).

Interventions. As the description of the cycle suggests, all the interventions exercised in controlling and managing a single aggressive episode are also appropriate in managing the early phases of cyclical aggression. The key difference is the role that countertransference feelings play (Giovacchini 1989; Maier et al. 1987, 1988; Sandler et al. 1970b). These feelings become the limiting factor in the ability of the staff to continue to provide humane care. Consequently, it is the responsibility of the administrator of the facility and of the staff themselves to recognize the presence of these feelings and to provide a mechanism whereby they can be resolved (Lakovics 1984; Mendota Mental Health Institute 1989a). The staff must be well trained in aggression management skills with well-designed seclusion rooms available and appropriate chemical restraints. They also need to know that their immediate supervisors and senior administrators understand their feelings and are willing to give them the opportunity to express and resolve these feelings.

When staff are able to process their feelings as they develop, instead of remaining fearful or angry at the patients and therefore distancing themselves from them, they develop the healthy, martial arts concept of "safe distance" (Westbrook and Ratti 1980). This means that they have given themselves the right to work safely with the patients. Consciousness has been raised. When this occurs, the staff and patient can develop trust because the staff no longer deny that at times they experience powerful negative feelings, and, therefore, these feelings no longer unconsciously govern the relationship. Trust becomes possible so that other appropriate forms of treatment can develop (Johansen 1983; Schroeder 1986).

Case Example and Discussion

A recently admitted female patient with a suspected diagnosis of schizophrenia began pacing up and down the corridor of a locked civil unit. By the time the staff had noticed the behavior and decided to assess the patient, she had begun yelling at patients in an indiscriminate manner while she appeared to be talking to unknown persons. One of the female staff walked out to contact the patient. As she walked up to the patient, the patient suddenly stepped toward her and yelled, "Get away from me, you slut!" Surprised, the staff member stepped back as the patient brushed by her. She followed the patient down the hall and motioned to the staff in the nursing station to come out to assist. The patient, who sensed she was being followed, turned around and yelled again. The staff member stopped, but this was not enough. The patient began yelling obscenities and began walking toward the staff member, who looked to see if help was coming from the nursing station. She could not see anyone. She quickly made a decision to see if the patient would respond to her voice. She did not know the patient's first name so she said, in a voice loud enough to catch the patient's attention but not so loud that it would frighten her, "Stop yelling. I'm not going to harm you. Stop." This seemed to catch the patient's attention and alerted the other staff because a staff member appeared in the corridor.

Meanwhile, the patient continued to escalate her behavior. She maintained her verbal attack on the female staff member and increased the intensity of her threats. The staff member tried again to talk to her, saying, "I hear you. I am not going to harm you." She could see three of her teammates moving slowly down the corridor toward them. The patient sensed their movement and turned sideways so she could see all staff.

It appeared as though the patient was calming down, but suddenly she yelled and lunged at the female staff member before her. The staff member stepped back and cushioned the force of the attack with her leg, but they both fell to the floor. Other staff joined them in seconds and after a minute of scuffling, the patient was subdued.

Now in control, the staff member gently told the patient, who was still yelling obscenities, to calm down. When it was clear she would not, the staff called for help and restrained and carried the patient to the seclusion room. The psychiatrist arrived just as the staff were going to leave the seclusion room. He did a quick assessment, agreed with the need for seclusion, and went to the nursing station to write the order. The staff then evacuated the seclusion room. The female staff member who was attacked discovered she had a sore elbow and a small cut on her face. The nursing supervisor agreed to send her to the medical clinic, where her injuries were assessed and treated. She returned to work the next day.

The following day, the psychiatrist, nurse, and safety officer who made up the aggression postmortem committee reviewed the incident and made the following report:

> *Description of the incident:* The talk down and seclusion of a female patient on the admission unit on January 7, 1993, was managed in a humane, ethical manner. The staff saw the preaggressive behavior (pacing, yelling) as potentially threatening. They sent one of the staff to assess the patient, who suddenly escalated from verbal abuse and threats to a physical assault on the staff. Although the staff member tried to talk the patient down, the patient appeared to be attending to internal stimuli and did not respond. Before the staff could assemble to take control of the patient in a more controlled manner, the patient attacked. The staff were forced to take the patient to the floor. One staff member was injured, sent to the clinic, and returned to work the next day. The patient was not injured. The incident was uneventful after the patient was placed in seclusion.
>
> *Recommendations:* 1) The patient had a history of sudden attack, especially on females. The history should have been available to the staff. 2) Because there did not appear to be any immediate risk to staff or other patients, the staff could have planned their intervention more carefully. The need for more help could have been considered. 3) The staff could have sent two members to assess the patient since there were three staff available at the time. 4) The injury was caused by the hard floor. The floors on the patient units in the admission building should be carpeted. 5) One staff member should be assigned to monitor all patient behavior in the dayroom and in the principal corridor. 6) Video surveillance might be a more cost-effective way to achieve the same goal. 7) Staff would benefit from a refresher course on talking down escalating patients.

The example and postmortem report are typical of countless aggressive incidents. Although the example may not be comprehensive, we think these comments are relevant. The example illustrates the usual sequence of events. The staff member did try to talk to the patient. She also tried to alert the other staff, who seemed to have forgotten about her mission. There were three staff present. This is one more than the staffing pattern at many facilities. There was a "plan." That is, they noticed the aberrant behavior and planned to assess it. The sudden attack is also typical. It is nearly impossible to tell when an agitated patient is going to attack. The best guide to prevention is to recognize that verbal abuse and verbal threats are clear signs that the process may escalate if not managed very carefully. This is not to fault the staff, because these incidents can change from controlled to out of control in a matter of seconds. The take down was in reality a "pile on." These are never pretty interventions. Staff know that and only expect that they will not be second-guessed about their performance after the event. Finally, reports like this one make administrators happy, but they can fail the staff. It may be the impersonal nature of such reports that has given them a bad name with line staff. Nevertheless, there is useful information in such reviews. Still, staff are often put off by the antiseptic quality of a typed report, which coldly outlines what was an intensely affect-laden event.

Transference and Countertransference

The psychiatric literature demonstrates that fear and anger are the most common countertransference reactions aroused in staff who work with aggressive patients (Colson et al. 1986; Lanza 1983). In fact, for staff who work with repetitively aggressive patients in closed systems such as inpatient units, fear and anger are the principal long-term occupational hazards of their work (Lanza 1985). It is not surprising that staff feel frightened and angry at patients who threaten (Fink 1990; Miller 1985), injure (Carmel and Hunter 1989), and even kill (Annis and Baker 1986; Turns and Gruenberg 1973) them. What is surprising is how frequently these feelings are left unaddressed or unchecked by the staff so that they become the driving force behind nearly every decision made regarding the patients. Perhaps it is because staff have significant difficulty tolerating strong feelings of fear, anger, helplessness, and frustration that the most common response is to deny the existence of these feelings (Sandler et al. 1970a). Because unresolved countertransference reactions have a significant impact on individual patient care, they are, in our opinion, the primary reason that the management of aggressive patients remains in the "dark side of psychiatry" (Lion 1987). Before we can properly understand how staff members react to aggressive patients, it is necessary to understand the stages involved in the escalating behavior of an agitated patient. The process of escalation described below is a more detailed description of the preaggression,

aggression, and control phases of the linear aggression sequence. This description focuses specifically on the patient's behavioral changes and associated feelings. It is intended to clarify how a patient escalating to aggression transfers feelings onto the target of this aggression.

The Process of Transference

The process that an aggressive patient may go through when escalating toward physical aggression can be divided into five stages (Table 7–1). These five behavioral stages include minor motor changes, verbal abuse or threats, major motor changes, physical aggression, and exhaustion. These stages are commonly associated with a range of patient feelings: anxiety or frustration, hostility, anger, rage, and relaxation. Not every patient experiences these feelings, and the feelings do not proceed in this order for every case. Nonetheless, the process of the behavioral stages and their associated feelings is common enough to be identified as the typical order of escalation that could result in physical aggression and control (Mendota Mental Health Institute 1989b). Physical aggression causes significant physiological arousal in patients or staff who may be the target of attack. The analytic concept transference (Van Rybroek and Maier 1987) has traditionally referred to unconscious feelings that originate from relationships that were significant in the patient's earlier life and then are transferred onto the therapist. This concept can be applied to the aggressive patient as well (Sandler et al.

Table 7–1. Stages of escalation

Patient behavioral stages	Patient associated feelings	Staff reactions
Minor motor	Anxiety/frustration	Empathy
Verbal abuse, verbal threats	Hostility	Anxiety
Major motor	Anger	Fear/anger
Physical aggression	Rage	Counteraggression
Exhaustion	Relaxation	Frustration (no tension, release)

Note. The aggressive patient passes through five behavioral stages in a typical aggression incident. There are specific feelings associated with each stage. Staff reactions vary with the stage of escalation.

1970d). Patients who are aggressive transfer their feelings (usually anger or rage) in a physical manner onto their victims. The escalating process of psychological arousal results in the physical projection, or transference, of the feelings onto the actual body of the victim.

With the above as a foundation, consider the typical reaction of staff to the five stages of escalation experienced by the patient. When the staff observe minor motor changes that may indicate feelings of anxiety and frustration, they approach the patient in an empathic manner. When the patient surprises staff by responding with verbal abuse or threats of physical harm, they respond by becoming anxious and concerned. Next, as the patient escalates to major motor behavior, the staff most typically feel fearful and in retrospect identify that it was at this stage when they began to feel anger. The very fact that the patient in this stage is pacing rapidly, invading other people's space, and making verbally abusive and threatening comments is alarming and frightening. If the patient escalates to actual physical aggression, the staff is empowered to contact that patient and subdue the patient if necessary. Feelings of self-preservation can be typical during this stage.

The counteraggression required to subdue a patient who is in the process of injuring or attempting to injure could jolt the staff member into the shocking awareness that he or she could become a killer in self-defense. The average clinician finds it very difficult to maintain this awareness. Nevertheless, aggression, if severe enough, can arouse murderous impulses in staff. The extreme discomfort accompanying the realization that one could become a killer given the right circumstances may account for the fact that staff often have such strong denial around the whole issue of managing patient aggression.

Once the aggressor is sufficiently controlled, exhausted, and perhaps beginning to relax, the staff are also able to relax physically. However, following aggression they will not be able to release the intense feelings aroused in them as a result of the physical experience. Typically they feel frustrated. The staff, therefore, go through a series of feeling changes as the stages of escalation progress, except they end where the patient began, frustrated.

As shown in Table 7–1, staff go through the feeling processes of empathy and then move to anxiety, fear/anger, and counteraggression and end with frustration. In a real sense, the staff reactions in their sequence trail behind the patient's feelings, making it plausible to postulate that the patient's feelings are transferred to staff when the staff become the target of the aggression. Staff who experience this feeling chain repeatedly, without a means of support, will in turn develop chronic countertransference reactions. All too often the psychological reactions of staff to each single aggression are minimized. By minimizing the impact of aggression on staff, a subtle denial takes place that ultimately will handicap staff in their development of effective approaches to the prevention, management, and treatment of aggressive behavior. If the staff are consumed by unresolved feelings of fear and anger toward patients, they will not be able to see clearly how to develop more humane and effective interventions (Cornfield and Fielding 1980).

A Countertransference Policy and Procedure

To identify and work through countertransference feelings resulting from aggression, it is incumbent on psychiatric facilities to have a policy governing the process for all levels of staff. The policy should derive from a study of incidents of aggression events (Depp 1976; Lion and Reid 1983; Silver and Yudofsky 1987; Sparr 1989) and result in a description of characteristics of repetitive aggressors (Barber et al. 1988). Emphasis should be given to the current intervention strategies that favor the least-restrictive alternative but are, nevertheless, safe (Glynn et al. 1989; Infantino and Musingo 1985). The facility should state its intent to protect staff and patients by stubbornly developing a humane environment (Gunderson 1978) that minimizes risk (Drummond et al. 1989). Finally, the policy must be supported by the top administrative staff because they realize the significant impact aggression can have on the ability of staff to provide humane care (Lehmann et al. 1983). The policy should be explained to all new employees and should include the following basic information:

1. Working with aggressive patients will at times arouse intense personal feelings of fear and anger, among other feelings (Brown 1980; Giovacchini 1989; Groves 1978; Strasburger 1987).

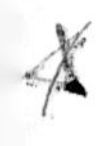

2. Staff are *expected to* identify and share these feelings with their peers and supervisor (Boyer 1979; Epstein 1979; Giovacchini 1979; Marshall 1979).
3. The clinical administration will provide four forums where these feelings can be discussed: during development of patient treatment

plans, at team meetings, during Me-Time, and during individual supervision.

4. Should these feelings cause a change in the ability to provide humane treatment to a patient, staff will be expected to address the issues that prevent them from delivering humane care. The personnel process may be utilized to shape the required change, including referral to the employee assistance program.
5. If, over time, a staff member is unable to manage feelings such as fear and anger, and it is noticeable in work performance, there may be an expectation to change work areas.

Having four forums where these feelings can be processed, staff are encouraged and shaped to develop greater skill in dealing with their feelings. Further, in the structure called Me-Time (Maier 1986), discussed at length later, they are given permission to describe how they feel about the patients in any manner that they find satisfying for their emotional needs (Sandler et al. 1970b).

Stages of the Countertransference Process

The stages of escalation describe the feeling process of an individual aggression episode. When an individual episode of aggression multiplies to repeated aggressions, a different intrapsychic countertransference process evolves. Figure 7–3 illustrates a six-stage sequence in the evolution of countertransference feelings as they move from acceptable conscious awareness to unconscious denial and acting out. These stages are discernibly different and indicate a growing intensity of feeling that progressively challenges the psychological defenses of the staff.

Figure 7–3 shows the means by which the visible signs of each stage are assessed by the individual staff member and others. Glancing down to "personal intervention," it can be seen that in the initial stages simple personal assessment or awareness of the development of negative feelings is sufficient to manage them. But as the feelings intensify and strain the individual psychological defense system, it may be that peers and other staff as well as the supervisor are required to assist in managing feelings too weighty to be handled alone (Winnicott 1949). Finally, if the above interventions fail and the feelings grow in intensity and complexity, personal therapy may be in order as a means to offer resolution and holistic self-acceptance (Wilber 1981).

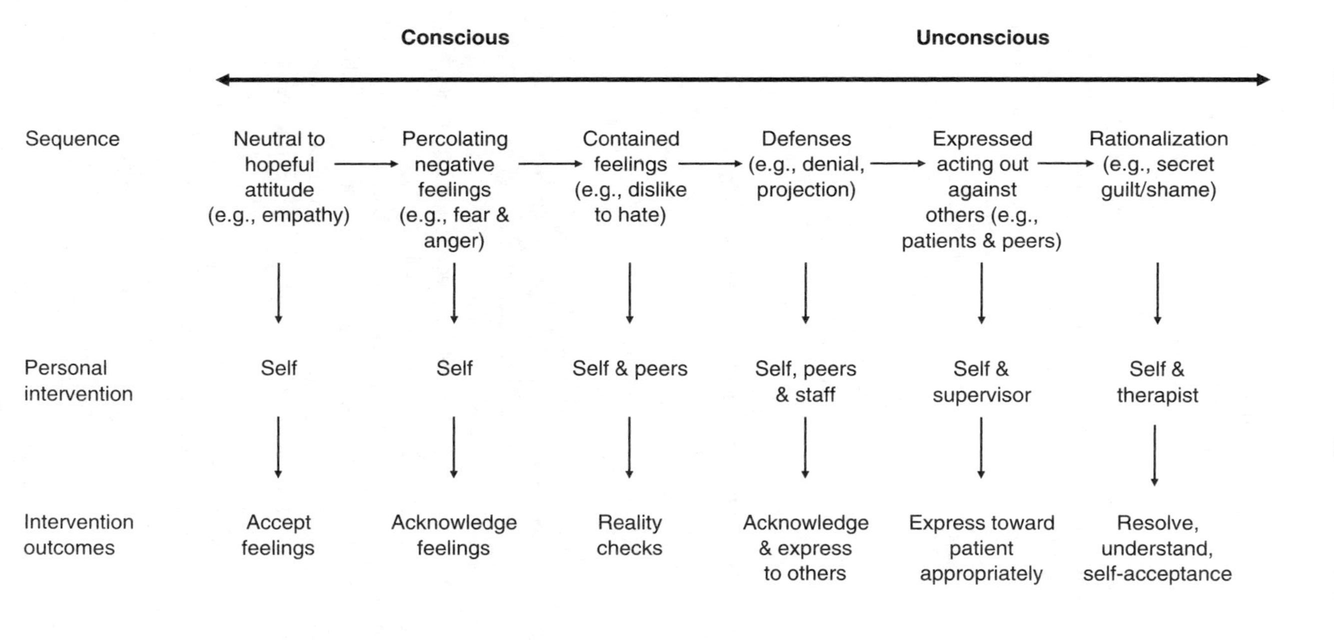

Figure 7–3. Countertransference stages.

Countertransference sequence: neutral to hopeful attitude. Most staff members bring a neutral to hopeful or empathic attitude to their first encounter with a patient. The initial interview (Mackinnon 1980) can be revealing. Often, significant information about the patient and about the staff surfaces. Typically in the first encounter, staff are less judgmental and more tolerant and, when emotionally challenged, less vulnerable. The original innocence of the first encounter usually reveals an acceptance of a broad range of feelings about the patient. Sometimes, of course, there is an immediate acceptance or rejection of the patient because of personal factors (e.g., the patient reminds the staff person of a significant other). In such situations, the staff person may be aware of the emergence of the second stage, "percolating" feelings. When intense (and usually negative) feelings such as fear or anger soar into consciousness, immediate self-management is required.

Countertransference sequence: percolating feelings. In the more typical situation, especially during the "honeymoon phase" of relationships with difficult patients, feelings generated in the initial encounter are more likely to appear slowly. The staff get to know the true nature of the patient. These feelings can be viewed as percolating, more or less bubbling up a bit at a time.

When this process begins, the staff person, in becoming aware that feelings are there, may not be able to manage them in a satisfactory manner. Full acceptance is a rare occurrence. This is not surprising because the very fact that the feelings are percolating may not be a reflection of a direct relationship between the staff person and the patient's stimulus. Rather, percolating feelings bubble up into awareness because they tend to be unmanageable within the staff member's own defense system, and the patient acts as a stimulus to activate unconscious feelings in the staff member, earned in previous relationships.

In the best case scenario, the percolating feelings are fully accepted. More often than not, the nature of the feelings and the interplay of personal factors signal that full acceptance will take time. But their full acknowledgment can be brought forth and recognized. A healthy resolution at this stage is for the staff person to acknowledge that a patient is generating intense feelings that are difficult to accept and integrate fully.

Countertransference sequence: feeling containment. As countertransference feelings grow in intensity, the staff person may have difficulty acknowledging them, which is the principal means of managing them. Often there is a struggle in the psyche to contain the strong feelings in a conscious, and then not so conscious, manner. In the third stage of feeling, containment, staff members can no longer count on self-assessment of feelings because a significant part of themselves cannot tolerate or even cognitively acknowledge the feelings. Conscious containment becomes the best mode of coping. Although the staff person consciously tries to cope by not expressing or acting on negative feelings, such a personal management approach may not be completely successful. Reality checks with peers about the feelings may validate their existence because of the more objective perceptions of another person. Reality checks from peers can be the feedback that the current self-management strategy is effective or that another coping response should be pursued.

Unconscious defenses are in play all the time. Obviously, when containment is the chief method of coping, the feelings are beyond the healthiest psychological checks and balances. It is not difficult to see that more exposure to the patient in an unmodified context will result in a further evolution of the countertransference process. The strength of the countertransference feeling aroused will begin to press more fully into unconscious psychological defenses.

Feeling containment can be explained by imagining that a staff person is like a "vase" with a finite capacity for holding feelings. As the staff members move from one day to the next, they will ultimately "fill up" on their feelings. Once feelings rise to the level of the vase's lip, there is nowhere else for them to go but "out." Therefore, staff contain feelings as long as they can, and then their unconscious has to find a way to release them. The release may occur through direct or indirect ways. It may occur at work against peers or patients or somewhere in their personal life. Regardless, release of negative feelings will take place once the staff can no longer contain them by maintaining a healthy intrapsychic balance.

Countertransference sequence: unconscious defenses. For reasons that are unclear, denial and projection are the unconscious defenses that tend to be activated when powerful countertransference reactions build up. If the first mechanism, denial, could be translated into words, the following might be stated, "Yes, I am frightened by this patient, and I've tried to put it out of my mind because I don't like that feeling. Although I know on some level that this patient frightens me, I've contained that feeling so well that I no longer feel it. Therefore, I don't feel frightened because there no longer is anything to frighten me." Because, by definition, psychological defenses are unconscious, it is quite likely that denial is in operation in such cases. The danger in this progression is the false sense of security resulting from a feeling that is felt no longer but nonetheless is "known" at some level. When our feelings become blocked through this powerful denial mechanism, our normal alert system to dangerous aspects of our environment is significantly impaired.

In the defense of projection, the staff person attributes his or her own fear to the patient in a way that could be translated into words such as, "Yes, I used to be frightened of this patient, but now I can see that he is actually more afraid of me than anything else. Therefore he is pretty weak, and I don't have to be concerned about him." Because of this projection, the fear in the staff person can no longer act as an alerting mechanism when the patient might really be threatening aggression. When staff fear is projected onto the patient as though the patient actually is the one who is frightened, the staff person, at the least, will be set up to mismanage the patient and, at the most, will exacerbate aggression.

It is at this stage that the concept of "Me-Time" becomes operational. During this specially designated time during the workday, the staff members are expected to pour out some of their feeling contents so as to drain off emotions that will negatively impact on their work performance. If staff openly express themselves during these meetings and receive feedback from peers, their conscious awareness of feelings may reappear. In this way, defenses such as denial and projection can be identified, and staff have the opportunity not only to experience the release of contained emotions, but also to reintroduce more effective coping mechanisms.

Countertransference sequence: acting out. The entrance of unconscious mechanisms often is first recognized when the acting-out behavior that inevitably accompanies them results in patient mismanagement or patient abuse. Acting out (Sandler et al. 1970c) can be observed in several different ways. Complaints by the patients about particular staff may increase. Other staff may note the unhealthy nature of the relationship and try to intervene. In the worst case scenario, actual patient abuse is witnessed, and other staff are obligated to report the behavior.

When this occurs, the supervisor and possibly other authorities must become involved (Merkel and Pillard 1987). Informal or formal discussions with peers and other staff are no longer sufficient. The supervisor must review the relevant data but with a focus on the countertransference process with the staff member. When this is done in a professional way, the staff member should be able to identify his or her feelings, share them with the supervisor, and finally express them in an appropriate manner.

The supervisor, of course, may discover that the acting-out behavior arises not just from the interaction with the patient, but from other staff dynamics or personal issues such as family problems or alcohol abuse. When other factors appear to be involved, a referral to an employee assistance program or to a counselor may be necessary. The key to this type of referral will likely arise from the assessment not only that the staff member has other personal problems connected to poor work performance, but that he or she minimizes these problems as well. Overuse of rationalizations as an explanation for acting-out behaviors is a common way this process can be recognized.

Countertransference sequence: rationalization. Facing limits in oneself is difficult for all persons, including those with professional training (Maier et al. 1989). When rationalizations or other similar explanations are overused to minimize the impact of one's inappropriate behavior toward patients (or others), the threshold for personal therapy has been met. The most common time for staff to begin a rationalizing process is when they have made a particularly punitive response to an "unsavory" patient. Staff may secretly feel guilt about their acting out on a patient but will not easily let go of a harsh decision without intervention. The principal intervention question is "What is this patient's behavior doing to my decision-making ability?" If there are no frank discussions among staff about how their feelings impact on their decisions, a chronic pattern of decision making, based on powerful countertransference reactions, will take place. This may result in anything from a perpetual bad attitude, to patient abuse. It is possible, with supervision, that staff could adopt the viewpoint that the most difficult patients are the ones who will "teach" them the most about their personal deficits. With such a perspective, staff members can gain a better understanding about themselves as well as provide better patient care.

Consideration also must be given to the fact that some staff do not have the interpersonal skills to work with patients who elicit strong negative feelings. For some staff, no amount of intervention would appropriately diffuse negative countertransference reactions. It may be well known to everyone working with a particular staff person that he or she simply does not appear able to cope emotionally with a specific patient. The best guidance there is to counsel the staff to identify these deficits so they can, at a minimum, respond to them in a neutral manner. The fact is that some staff are better at working with some patients than others. When staff cannot resolve negative countertransference issues and the maladaptive behavior that results from them, it may be time to discuss transfer to a less-intense environment or, if severe enough, consider termination.

Me-Time: The Process of Resolution

Me-Time in Context

Every effort must be made to encourage staff to learn how to understand and attenuate the process of escalating aggressive behavior and to work through the stages of countertransference that result from it (Heider 1985). The process of resolving these feelings begins with a conscious awareness that countertransference exists. This is tantamount to saying that the denial generally associated with this process has been consciously acknowledged and that a full-faced attempt to prevent and resolve countertransference feelings through ongoing discussions is expected and valued. The discussions are sanctioned to occur on an informal and formal basis (Monroe et al. 1988).

The informal discussion occurs throughout the day by all levels of staff. These are dialogues that occur in the corridor, nursing station, staff break room (but away from the patients), at lunch, and after work. In these discussions, the staff simply acknowledge how they feel toward individual patients or toward the whole patient group. These discussions are invaluable and establish a general climate that will legitimize all types of feelings, good and bad, from hate to love.

However, as informal discussions, they can hardly be effective in bringing intransigent countertransference reactions into awareness so they can be resolved. Their worth is in laying the groundwork for a semiformal process called Me-Time.

Me-Time is a regularly scheduled semisupervisory session that occurs between all levels of staff under the direction of the unit supervisor(s). Me-Time is recommended to take place a minimum of 1 hour per week but up to 1 hour per day on units with a high rate of aggression. In general, the goal of Me-Time is to tune in consciously to the feeling processes of staff. It may be a difficult process in itself and will likely be met with the typical resistances such as silence, anger, projection, and rationalization. When staff are allowed to meet in a confidential manner on a regular basis, however, a process will evolve in which staff will come to trust each other enough to share their real feelings. There are only a few simple rules. All nursing and clinical staff must attend. Racist and sexist comments are not acceptable. Staff are encouraged to express themselves in language that is meaningful and satisfying to them. They may talk about individual patients, the current patient group, their peers, their own idiosyncratic issues, or anything else that may be on their minds. The process of encouraging free expression and working through staff differences when life and death are at stake is beyond the scope of this chapter.

A typical example of the process of a Me-Time is that of resolving staff splitting (Gabbard 1989) about the management and treatment approach for a patient. In this scenario, staff feelings are polarized in which one group wants to approach the patient as heartless "hard hats" who "act like Nazis"; the other group, the "bleeding hearts," wants to approach the patient "like forgiving Nuns." These polar opposite approaches toward the patient can be very difficult to resolve unless the supervisor understands that time is needed to allow the staff to reconcile their differences. Staff cannot be protected from the process of their own struggle. Instead, the supervisor should allow a struggle to take place. With proper regulation, the supervisor should encourage the staff to express the range of their opposed feelings. This sometimes painful process will move toward the resolving phase where reasonable management decisions result. Understanding that the affect has collected in the polarities of the staff, and that it is imperative that it be discharged before any risk-taking decisions are made, becomes the processing step for the staff.

Me-Time: How It Works

The first step of resolution, therefore, is to allow both sides to express themselves as completely as possible. After this catharsis, the silent majority usually begin to temper the polar positions and lead toward some central position. Through the work of the unit supervisors and those staff who are not as emotionally aroused, a compromise position can be established. Because risks need to be taken with patients who have been aggressive, the compromise position is the most reasonable position that the staff feeling will allow to occur, given the strength of the polar feelings. Such decision making is called "taking a reasonable risk." The concept of reasonable risk taking means that decisions are not made from feelings but from reason. Most important, however, is the philosophy that before any decisions are made about aggressive patients, all staff are given the opportunity to free themselves of emotions that would only cloud good decision making.

On occasion, informal and semiformal processes of working through countertransference cannot impact on the intensity of the countertransference that an individual staff person may feel. In situations such as this, the countertransference must be addressed in the most formal forum, that of individual supervision. In this forum, the individual supervisor will have an opportunity to discuss the work performance of the staff member as it relates to the staff member's feelings for selected patients. The supervisor also can make an assessment of issues that may be unresolved in the staff's personal life that may be appearing at work. It is not uncommon for staff who are experiencing stress in their personal life to act it out at work. Once the work performance has been properly assessed, the supervisor can suggest appropriate ways for the employee to make corrections in the work area. The supervisor may also need to refer the individual to the employee assistance program for further counseling. At times it may be appropriate for a supervisor to suggest that the employee seek private counseling and even therapy.

The multifaceted approach described above of informal, semiformal, and formal ways of addressing countertransference issues complies with the goals of an established countertransference policy and can greatly contribute to an environment free of patient abuse. It also may be the key ingredient to help staff remain emotionally healthy while working with potentially aggressive patients (Minkoff and Stern 1985; Tardiff 1989).

Case Example and Discussion

The staff of an inpatient unit serving acute patients expressed concern to the unit supervisor about a recently admitted patient who had been manifesting some symptoms of agitation and hostility toward patients and staff. In the Friday afternoon team meeting, they worried that the patient would continue to escalate and become more problematic over the weekend. The supervisor politely listened to them but ultimately stated that they were "overconcerned" about this patient and that no special precautions needed to be taken. By Friday evening, the patient had challenged several patients to fight him and had been verbally abusive to staff. Although everyone was on alert to potential problems, no plan had been established to de-escalate the situation. During the lunch hour on Saturday, when the unit was minimally staffed, the patient became very hostile and started to threaten everyone. The staff attempted to talk him down but he refused to comply with their redirection. The patient continued to escalate. In response, a disorganized and understaffed take down was attempted. In the fracas, the charge nurse received a broken nose, and one of the aide staff suffered a sprained back.

On Monday, the busy unit supervisor arrived for the regularly scheduled Me-Time knowing that the staff would be angry about the aggression on the weekend. The supervisor opened the meeting by ignoring the pressing feelings and started to tell the staff about some concerns raised by the dietary department. The staff, well acquainted with the process of Me-Time, stopped the supervisor because they wanted to talk about the recent aggression and staff injuries. The supervisor, in an attempt to deflect the discussion away from the feeling level, tried to switch the discussion to the patient's diagnosis, so they could formulate a modified treatment plan. The staff, however, persisted in discussing their feelings about how in the Friday meeting they had expressed serious concerns about the patient's preaggression symptoms and how the supervisor had dismissed the need for preventive action. They expressed anger at the supervisor for dismissing their input during Friday's meeting and for appearing unconcerned about the injury to the staff.

After several attempts to deny and deflect the feelings, the supervisor realized and admitted that the staff reactions to the way the situation was managed were legitimate. The discussion then progressed to how the staff felt the supervisor did not give them enough input into the management of potentially serious circumstances involving patient and staff safety. The staff reported that they felt disrespected because the supervisor did not trust their judgment about patients. The supervisor responded that he felt very accountable for the care of patients and therefore could not relinquish his responsibility easily. In further discussion, the supervisor and the staff carefully walked through the decision-making process of the last aggression and considered how the incident could have been managed better. The staff stated that they were willing to work together with the supervisor about these important issues but that the supervisor had to do a better job taking their concerns seriously. The staff pointed out that the supervisor actually would be more responsible if he trusted them more and acted on some of their suggested interventions.

This typical but somewhat idealized example illustrates several important points. Managing inpatient aggression requires multidisciplinary skills, those of line staff and those of the trained clinician. Respectful communication is essential between all levels of staff and is the best way to prevent aggression. Although it is always easy to second-guess decisions, in the above case the principal decision maker, the unit supervisor (who could be a psychiatrist or psychologist, for example), made an effort to listen to the staff concerns but failed to solicit specific reasons or specific precautions before labeling their fears as an "overconcern." Learning how to identify the behaviors of a potentially aggressive patient, which may reliably contribute to a plan of prevention, from the feelings staff have that they are at risk is critical in the preaggression phase. The aggression postmortem should pick up this dissonance and suggest guidelines that could result in better communication between the levels of staff.

The example cannot describe in a detailed way the replay of the whole process. This Me-Time, however, did give the line staff an opportunity to vent their anger toward one of their "superiors." These staff members are always at the bottom of the authority-power hierarchy. Yet they often have good ideas and exercise good judgment when faced with unpredictable circumstances. It is important that they feel supported. Although it may even be true that one or more of the staff have a tendency to overreact in such situations (which is not suggested in the example), this is the kind of issue that other staff members might bring up. The staff usually will not support each other if they themselves believe that a patient was provoked into self-defense because the staff member had a need to overcontrol the patient. At the same time, the supervisors are not always on the hot seat. In fact, most often they are in a position to relieve staff-staff impasses. They are often the power brokers who can help shape staff opinion, practice, or values. Me-Time then becomes an in-service for all staff members and an opportunity for healing staff splitting. Team building is an important part of the process. Although every Me-Time is not a charged, emotional encounter, the very fact that the opportunity is there, on a regularly scheduled basis, lets all levels of staff know that they do not need to wait for a crisis to express their concerns to their supervisors or to each other. This is the principal strength of Me-Time.

Summary

Managing the intense reactions that are a natural response to aggressive behavior is difficult, at best, for all levels of staff that work in inpatient settings. Before staff can rationally plan to identify and work through these intense emotions, they must come to know and understand the processes that produce them. The model presented at the beginning of the chapter is a first step at describing the phases of aggression. Understanding these phases makes it possible to focus more intensely on the specific process of escalation. This process is the one that carries the energy transfer from the patient to the staff. Staff members are emotionally traumatized by each aggressive event. The accumulation of unresolved "negative" emotion factors into the way staff members relate to patients. Recognizing this fact leads to the formulation of the dynamics of aggression cycles. Unresolved staff countertransference feelings govern the rhythm of aggression on many inpatient units, despite significant and variable psychopathology in the patient.

Understanding that the accumulation of unresolved countertransference feelings plays a significant role in defining the humane quality of the environment of the unit makes it incumbent on those in charge of the hospital to develop methods to prevent and work through such feelings. Some form of policy or training will need to be developed. A countertransference policy and procedure and the structure called

Me-Time are the two clinical and administrative responses that address these concerns. There are many other aspects of aggression management that are relevant to this issue, but the interventions described above are necessary elements in any comprehensive approach in the management of staff feelings to aggressive patients and for subsequent efficacy as well as safety of the clinical staff.

References

Adler G: Helplessness in the helpers. Br J Med Psychol 45:315–326, 1972

Alaron RD, Bancroft AA, Daniels TD: Dynamics of the inpatient psychiatric setting. Psychiatric Annals 18:102–105, 1988

American Psychiatric Association: Diagnostic and Statistical Manual of Mental Disorders, 4th Edition. Washington, DC, American Psychiatric Association, 1994

Annis LV, Baker CA: A psychiatrist's murder in a mental hospital. Hosp Community Psychiatry 37:505–506, 1986

Barber JW, Hundley P, Kellog E, et al: Clinical and demographic characteristics of 15 patients with repetitively assaultive behavior. Psychiatr Q 59:213–224, 1988

Binder RL: The use of seclusion on an inpatient intervention unit. Hosp Community Psychiatry 30:266–269, 1979

Binder RL, McCoy SM: A study of patient's attitudes toward placement in seclusion. Hosp Community Psychiatry 34:1052–1054, 1983

Boyer LB: Countertransference with severely regressed patients, in Countertransference. Edited by Epstein L, Feiner A. New York, Jason Aronson, 1979, pp 347–373

Brown LF: Staff countertransference reactions in the hospital treatment of borderline patients. Psychiatry 43:333–345, 1980

Carmel H, Hunter M: Staff injuries from inpatient violence. Hosp Community Psychiatry 40:41–46, 1989

Colson DB, Allen JG, Coyne L, et al: An anatomy of countertransference: staff reactions to difficult psychiatric hospital patients. Hosp Community Psychiatry 47:923–928, 1986

Cornfield RB, Fielding SD: Impact of the threatening patient on ward communications. Am J Psychiatry 137:616–619, 1980

Depp FC: Violent behavior patterns on psychiatric wards. Aggressive Behavior 2:295–306, 1976

Drummond DJ, Sparr LF, Gordon GH: Hospital violence reduction among high-risk patients. JAMA 26:2531–2534, 1989

Dubin WR: Emergency Psychiatry for the House Officer. Jamaica, NY, Spectrum Publications, 1985

Epstein L: The therapeutic function of hate in the countertransference, in Countertransference. Edited by Epstein L, Feiner A. New York, Jason Aronson, 1979, pp 213–234

Fink DL: Threats and assaults against residents. Paper presented at the 143rd annual meeting of the American Psychiatric Association, New York, May 14, 1990

Gabbard GO: Splitting in hospital treatment. Am J Psychiatry 144:444–451, 1989

Giovacchini PL: Countertransference with primitive mental states, in Countertransference. Edited by Epstein L, Feiner A. New York, Jason Aronson, 1979, pp 235–265

Giovacchini PL: Countertransference Triumphs and Catastrophes. New York, Jason Aronson, 1989

Glynn SM, Bowen LL, Marshall BD Jr, et al: Compliance with less restrictive aggression-control procedures. Hosp Community Psychiatry 40:82–84, 1989

Groves JE: Taking care of the hateful patient. N Engl J Med 298:883–887, 1978

Gunderson JG: Defining the therapeutic processes in psychiatric milieus. Psychiatry 41:327–335, 1978

Harris GT, Varney GW: Assaults and Assaulters in Psychiatric Facilities. New York, Grune & Stratton, 1983

Heider J: The Tao of Leadership. New York, Bantam Books, 1985

Infantino JA, Musingo S: Assaults and injuries among staff with and without training in aggression control techniques. Hosp Community Psychiatry 36:1312–1314, 1985

Johansen KH: The impact of patients with chronic character pathology on a hospital inpatient unit. Hosp Community Psychiatry 43:842–846, 1983

Kaplan SG, Wheeler EG: Survival skills for working with potentially violent clients. Am J Psychiatry 130:616–619, 1980

Kaplan SG, Wheeler EG: Survival skills for working with potentially violent clients: social casework. Journal of Contemporary Social Work, June, 1983, pp 339–346

Lakovics M: A classification of countertransference phenomena and its application to inpatient psychiatry. Psychiatr J Univ Ottawa 10:132–138, 1984

Lanza ML: The reactions of nursing staff to physical assault by a patient. Hosp Community Psychiatry 43:44–47, 1983

Lanza ML: How nurses react to patient assault. J Psychosoc Nurs Ment Health Serv 23:6–11, 1985

Lehmann LS, Padilla M, Clark S, et al: Training personnel in the prevention and management of violent behavior. Hosp Community Psychiatry 34:40–43, 1983

Lion JR: Evaluation and Management of the Violent Patient. Springfield, IL, Charles C Thomas, 1972

Lion JR: Training for battle: thoughts on managing aggressive patients. Hosp Community Psychiatry 38:882–884, 1987

Lion JR, Pasternak SA: Countertransference reactions to violent patients. Am J Psychiatry 130:207–210, 1980

Lion JR, Reid WH (eds): Assaults Within Psychiatric Facilities. New York, Grune & Stratton, 1983

Mackinnon RA: Psychiatric interview, in Comprehensive Textbook of Psychiatry/III, 3rd Edition, Vol 2. Edited by Kaplan HI, Freedman AM, Sadock BJ. Baltimore, MD, Williams & Wilkins, 1980, pp 895–905

Madden DJ, Lion JR: Rage, Hate, Assault and Other Forms of Violence. New York, Spectrum Publications, 1976

Maier GJ: Relationship security: the dynamics of keepers and kept. Journal for Science 31:603–608, 1986

Maier GJ, Van Rybroek GJ: Offensive images: managing aggression isn't pretty. Hosp Community Psychiatry 41:357, 1990

Maier GJ, Stava LJ, Morrow BR, et al: A model for understanding and managing cycles of aggression among psychiatric patients. Hosp Community Psychiatry 31:603–608, 1987

Maier GJ, Van Rybroek GJ, Doren DM, et al: A comprehensive model for understanding and managing aggressive inpatients. American Journal of Continuing Education in Nursing, Section C, 1988, pp 1–16

Maier GJ, Bernstein MJ, Musholt EA: Personal coping mechanisms for prison clinicians. Journal of Prison and Jail Health 8:29–39, 1989

Marshall RJ: Countertransference with children and adolescents, in Countertransference. Edited by Epstein L, Feiner A. New York, Jason Aronson, 1979, pp 407–441

McGee JJ: Gentle teaching. New Zealand Journal of Mental Retardation 40:13–24, 1985

Mendota Mental Health Institute: General Policy #22, Countertransference Issues, Forensic Center, Policy Manual. Madison, WI, Mendota Mental Health Institute, 1989a

Mendota Mental Health Institute: Interventions for Aggression, Training Program. Madison, WI, Mendota Mental Health Institute, 1989b

Merkel WT, Pillard CA: Applying modern management principles to clinical administration of a behaviorally oriented inpatient unit. Hosp Community Psychiatry 38:153–159, 1987

Miller RD: The harassment of forensic psychiatrists outside of court. Bull Am Acad Psychiatry Law 13:337–343, 1985

Minkoff K, Stern R: Paradoxes faced by residents being trained in the psychosocial treatment of people with chronic schizophrenia. Hosp Community Psychiatry 36:859–864, 1985

Monahan J: The Clinical Prediction of Violent Behavior. Rockville, MD, US Department of Health and Human Services, 1981

Monroe CM, Van Rybroek GJ, Maier GJ: Decompressing aggressive inpatients: breaking the aggression cycle to enhance positive outcome. Behavioral Sciences and the Law 6:543–557, 1988

Perls FS: Ego, Hunger and Aggression. New York. Vintage Books, 1947

Rada RT: The violent patient: rapid assessment and management. Psychosomatics 33:101–109, 1981

Sandler J, Dare C, Holder A: Basic psychoanalytic concepts, III: transference. Br J Psychiatry 116:667–672, 1970a

Sandler J, Holder A, Dare C: Basic psychoanalytic concepts, IV: countertransference. Br J Psychiatry 117:83–88, 1970b

Sandler J, Holder A, Dare C: Basic psychoanalytic concepts, VI: acting out. Br J Psychiatry 117:329–334, 1970c

Sandler J, Dare C, Holder A: Basic psychoanalytic concepts, VIII: special forms of transference. Br J Psychiatry 117:561–568, 1970d

Schroeder PJ: Recognizing transference and countertransference. J Psychosoc Nurs Ment Health Serv 23:21–26, 1986

Silver JM, Yudofsky SC: Documentation of aggression in the assessment of the violent patient. Psychiatric Annals 17:375–384, 1987

Sparr LF: Incident reporting is key to managing violence in hospitals. Psychiatric Times, April 1989

Strasburger LH: Countertransference with psychopathic patients. Psychiatric News, November 1987

Tanke ED, Yesavage JA: Characteristics of assaultive patients who do and do not provide visible cues of potential violence. Am J Psychiatry 142:1409–1413, 1985

Tardiff K: Assessment and Management of Violent Patients. Washington, DC, American Psychiatric Press, 1989

Thackery M: Therapeutics for Aggression: Psychological/Physical Crisis Interventions. New York, Human Sciences Press, 1987

Turns DM, Gruenberg EM: An attendant is murdered: the state hospital responds. Psychiatr Q 47:487–494, 1973

Van Rybroek GJ, Maier GJ: Aggressive inmates: hitting critical components of management. Correct Care 1:7, 1987

Westbrook A, Ratti O: Akido and the Dynamic Sphere. Rutland, VT, Charles E Tuttle, 1980

Wilber K: No Boundary: Eastern and Western Approaches to Personal Growth. Boston, MA, New Science Library, 1981

Winnicott DW: Hate in the counter-transference. Int J Psychoanal 30:699–674, 1949

Yudofsky SC, Silver JM, Jackson W, et al: The Overt Aggression Scale for the objective rating of verbal and physical aggression. Am J Psychiatry 143:35–39, 1986

Chapter 8

Nursing Staff as Victims of Patient Assault

Marilyn Lewis Lanza, R.N., D.N.Sc., Sc.

Much of the literature on patient assault focuses on prediction and intervention strategies. Although enormously important, these efforts are unlikely to eliminate the problem. The rate of assault in hospitals reflects the increasing violence in society (Adler et al. 1983; Binder and McNeil 1986; Browner 1987; Carmel and Hunter 1989; Conn and Lion 1983; Hodgkinson et al. 1985; Ionno 1983; Lehmann et al. 1983; Reid et al. 1985; Soloff 1987; Steadman et al. 1978; Tardiff 1984; Tardiff and Koenigsberg 1985).

Our estimates of assault are also low. A pivotal question in designing any investigation is identifying assault incidents. Identifying assaults is a particularly difficult task and a very important one because accuracy of incident documentation determines the quality of the data and of course the validity of the conclusions. Unfortunately for study purposes and the depiction of clinical reality, it is well documented in the literature that assaults are vastly underreported (Brizer et al. 1988; D. Campbell, M. Purtell, N. Swanson, and D. Laramore, unpublished report, 1989; Lanza 1988b; Lion et al. 1981; Monahan 1989; Silver and Yudofsky 1987).

Brizer and colleagues (1988) observed in a careful study using videotaping that nearly all low-hostility and many high-hostility as-

Portions of this chapter are reprinted from Lanza ML: "Nurses as Patient Assault Victims: An Update, Synthesis, and Recommendations." *Archives of Psychiatric Nursing* 6:163–171, 1992. Copyright 1992 W. B. Saunders Company. Used with permission.

saults were not reported using conventional procedures. Campbell and colleagues (unpublished report, 1989) interviewed nursing staff on nonpsychiatric units such as medical units and those caring for geriatric patients and patients suffering from Alzheimer's disease. The nursing staff indicated that assaults were vastly underreported. Lion and colleagues (1981) estimated that 80% of assaults are not reported. Lanza (1988b) found that half of the victims ($N = 37$) in a 3-month pilot study said that they had had at least one unreported assault during the year. The estimates of unreported assaults per victim ranged from 3 to as high as 300 (Lanza 1988b). Typical of incidents not reported were punches, slaps, and pinches to the arm or breast (Lanza 1988b). Silver and Yudofsky (1987) showed a 34%–71% difference between conventional methods used by hospitals to document assault occurrences and that developed by their investigation. Their detailed analysis of aggressive behaviors omitted by hospital records revealed that they comprised all forms of violence—physical as well as verbal—and aggression of all levels of severity from dangerously severe to mild.

There are a variety of reasons given for the underreporting of assault. These include

1. The variable definition of *assault* (Lanza 1988b; Monahan 1989; Pearson et al. 1986); many assault victims felt that assault should be reported only if it was "sufficiently severe."
2. Differential attributions made to the patient about the degree of intent to commit harm (Lanza 1988b).
3. Staff inurement to assault (Lanza 1988b; Lion et al. 1981); "assaults are so common here" (Lanza 1988b).
4. Staff attitude that assault is to be expected since they work in a high-risk environment (Lanza 1988b); "being hit is part of the job."
5. Staff characteristics such as peer pressure not to report and differential reporting based on sex of the person assaulted (Lanza 1988b).
6. Fear of blame (Lion et al. 1981).
7. Excessive paperwork involved to report assault and not enough time to complete it (Lanza 1988b; Lion et al. 1981).
8. Varying quality of information; information on reports may be invalid if reports are completed by persons not witness to the event or when information is incomplete (Drinkwater 1982).

The difficulty in exploring the impact of assault on nursing staff is further complicated by what appears to be a pervasive attitude that we should look at assault only from the patient's perspective. To examine the problem more fully—that is, to include the staff perspective—is somehow "detrimental" to the patient (Lanza 1982). This one-sided or split view (or adversarial view) is seen when examining such notions as patients' versus staff rights in terms of safety. Patients' rights are feared threatened when safety measures are discussed (Mappes and Zembaty 1981) rather than the more global view that only when all are safe—patients and staff—can patients' treatment be maximized (Ulrich 1978). Staff who are worried about safety cannot be fully mentally available to their patients (Halleck 1974; Lanza 1982; Scalfani 1986).

Assaults to Staff

Assaults to staff are a common occurrence. Carmel and Hunter (1989) reported 16% of the nursing staff were assaulted in a 1-year period. Although most assaults do not result in life-threatening injuries, serious injuries do occur, such as severe sprains, lacerations, fractures, and head trauma (Carmel and Hunter 1989; Lanza 1983, 1988b). The most common site of injury is the head (Lanza et al. 1992).

It is easy to underestimate the impact of an assault because physical injury is the most common measure used to assess assault impact. In fact, victims report intense and residual emotional reactions to "minor" assaults and threats of assault. In my experience, it is the victim's perceived sense of vulnerability that seems to be a key factor. This sense of vulnerability is not necessarily at the conscious level, as is discussed later.

Staff Reactions to Assault

Patients who are violent are perceived by staff as among the most difficult to treat (Colson et al. 1985, 1986). Lanza (1983) conducted a descriptive exploratory study in which nurses reported various short-term (1 week or less) and long-term (longer than 1 week) reactions to patient assault, including family pressures for them to change jobs or leave nursing. Reactions of nurse victims included emotional, social, biophysiological, and cognitive responses (Table 8–1). There are indi-

Table 8–1. Victim reactions to patient assault

Emotional	Social	Biophysiological	Cognitive
Short-term			
Helplessness Irritability Fear of returning to the scene of the assault Feeling of resignation Depression Anger Anxiety Shock Disbelief Self-blame Dependency	Change in relationship with coworkers Difficulty returning to work Fear of other patients Feel sorry for the patient who hit them Should have done something to prevent the assault	Startle response Sleep pattern disturbance Soreness Headaches	Denial of thoughts about the assault Preoccupation with thinking about the assault Considering change in lifestyle, job change
Long-term			
Fear of patient who hit them	Feel sorry for the patient who hit them	Body tension Soreness	Anger toward authority Wanting protection by authority and from authority's criticisms

cations that some staff felt they would be overwhelmed if they allowed themselves to admit their feelings. Some stated that if they allowed themselves to experience feelings about the likelihood of assault, they would not be able to function. Others felt they had no right to react since being assaulted was part of the job; some indicated they expected to be hit, believing it was part of their employment. Staff who received the most severe injuries indicated less fear of the patient who had assaulted them than did staff who were less severely injured. The cognitive reactions are elaborated because of the rich data.

Short-Term Cognitive Reactions

Short-term cognitive reactions ranged widely from denial of any thoughts to preoccupation with the assault to consideration of job and professional changes as the result of the assault.

Denial and rationalization were reflected by statements such as "I don't want to think about this. In every adversity there are seeds of a better experience. I try to look on the positive side. I don't feel remorse or revenge. I look ahead, not back."

Preoccupation with the assault focused on self-blame and on psychological and somatic reactions to the assault. Self-blame appeared as an obsession with one or more of the following areas: reviewing the incident to see if the victim had missed any cues, thinking of better ways to restrain patients or handle the assault, and trying to understand why the assault occurred. Reflecting concern with their own reactions, many staff indicated preoccupation with their body image, the possibility of permanent side effects or damage from the injury, the need to be physically dependent on others because of injuries sustained, an increased sense of vulnerability, and their ability to return to work.

Although many respondents, as noted, accepted assault as part of the job, some thought about a different career. For instance, one said, "I want to change my career. I don't have to take this. They don't pay me enough to take this abuse."

Long-Term Cognitive Reactions

Similarly, a wide range of long-term thoughts were expressed. Some staff reported no long-term thoughts. Some continued to experience earlier cognitive reactions. A new concern was administrative support of staff victims.

Denial and rationalization were reflected in the following: "I considered [the injury] an accident since it happened as the result of the assault. The patient was confused. I forgive and forget easily. The patient was not in his right mind and not totally responsible. Later I got to know the patient and developed a good relationship."

Some still blamed themselves. "It was my own stupidity. I should have called for help sooner."

Some staff showed continued concern about long-term physical side effects and an increased sense of vulnerability—for instance, "Will my neck always bother me?" Some victims thought about the dangerousness of their work situations. They became extracautious and shared intuitive feelings with other nursing staff about which patients might be dangerous. They thought about self-defense courses.

Concern about administrative support was indicated by statements such as "I should be free to defend myself without fear of criticism or losing my job. There should be concern with staff, not just patient, rights." Some felt guilty at not pressing charges against the patient but felt they would receive little administrative support.

Further Evidence of Assault as a Staff Stressor

Lion and colleagues (1981) and Janoff-Bulman and Frieze (1983) reported similar findings about the intensity and variety of victim reactions. Bernstein (1981) similarly reported that patient assault was a very frightening experience to the therapists he surveyed and that they frequently employed denial as a defense mechanism. Lanza (1985b) again identified denial as a reaction to assault when staff rated their own experience as an assault victim as less severe than the experience of coworkers in a comparable incident. M. L. Lanza and H. Kayne (unpublished report, 1990) again confirmed the range and intensity of victim response. Browner (1987) reported that assault on staff was considered a serious source of job stress. Carmel and Hunter (1989) and Browner elaborated on physical injuries suffered by staff. The concern about degree of staff support in dealing with assault situations was identified by Browner. Cust (1986) also found that staff were concerned about the right not to be assaulted and that a prevailing attitude of the legal judicial system was "If you chose to work in a psychiatric hospital, you accept the risk you will be assaulted."

Nurses reported reactions lasting up to 1 year and often beyond the time they returned to work. Rix (1987) found no relation between assault on staff and absenteeism. This may be due to the fact that staff remain on duty even after injured to "cover the unit" (Cust 1986). This was again confirmed by Lanza and Kayne (unpublished report, 1990); assaulted staff did not leave work or returned to work before they had felt recovered.

Factors Related to the Reporting of Assault as a Stressor

A variety of factors may influence the intensity of the ability to acknowledge the stress produced by being assaulted. These include coping style, identification with one's profession, sex, and severity of injury.

Those staff who characteristically approach rather than avoid conflict were more able to acknowledge the impact of assault. (The assault experiences were the same for all subjects.) Staff who were able to acknowledge the effect of assault used defense mechanisms such as intellectualization, obsessive behaviors, and ruminative worrying (Lanza 1988c). Those who did not acknowledge the intensity of the assault typically employed defenses such as repression, denial, and rationalization (Lanza 1988c).

Those who more strongly identified with their profession as measured by length of work experience, educational background, and level of position (job) were able to acknowledge their reactions (Lanza 1988c).

Women more readily acknowledged the intensity of their reactions than did men (Lanza 1988c).

There is a suggestion that those who were most severely injured were less fearful of the patient who assaulted them than were staff who were more mildly injured (Lanza 1983).

Blame

Blame is a particularly important concept when addressing the issue of patient assault. Almost everyone involved attributes blame. The victim often blames himself or herself and/or those in authority. Coworkers, albeit unwittingly, blame the assaulted. Those in authority or the "system" as a whole often engage in the process of blaming the victim (Ryan 1976).

This latter part of the blaming triangle is particularly important to understand because it has profound effects on increasing the incidence of patient violence. Simply stated, if an institution assumes that fault or responsibility lies with the assaulted staff member, then the institution can deny that there is a more general problem of patient assault. As a result, there is no determination of the extent of the problem of assault or recognition that a problem even exists. The assault of a staff member is seen as a rare occurrence and due to some unique characteristic in that person. The bottom line is that no prevention or intervention strategies are established to cope with the problem of assault, and the mythical reality is maintained that "we do not have a problem."

Current research on blame for assault has particularly important implications for the clinical situation. First and most importantly, blame for an event is not objectively determined (Lanza 1983, 1984a, 1987).

People give different interpretations to the same event based on their own personal views and characteristics. For example, the degree of blame made to a nurse victim for a patient assault is influenced by several factors. The age of the person making the judgment is the first factor (Lanza 1983, 1984a, 1987). The older the rater the more likely he or she will blame the victim.

The second factor is the judge's own experience as an assault victim (Lanza 1984a). That is, if a person has been assaulted in the past by a patient, that person is much less likely to blame another staff victim than would a person who has never been assaulted. Possibly, an experience as an assault victim has shattered the myth that assault does not happen or that fault necessarily lies with the victim.

The third factor is the sex of the victim (Lanza 1987, 1991). Women victims receive higher degrees of blame than do men.

The fourth factor is the severity of the assault (Lanza 1987, 1991). A very interesting observation is that victims who receive more minor injuries receive higher degrees of blame than victims who receive more severe injuries.

Preliminary data suggest no differences between staff who are assaulted and those who are not, other than position in the administrative hierarchy and time spent in direct patient contact (Lanza et al. 1992).

Wortman (1976) suggested that there is a nearly universal need to engage in blame when there is an untoward occurrence. Blaming allows one to feel safe and have control over the environment. Further, people function under an illusion of freedom in which they have control over their environment and are free of external influences. Wortman postulated that it may be painful or difficult to blame oneself or others for unfortunate outcomes, but it may be more painful to view the world as a place where undesirable events happen to innocent people on a random basis. As a result, although a clinician may not want to engage in the blaming process, it may be very difficult not to do so. Making this a conscious process that is open to staff discussion allows for a more productive approach.

Role Conflict

Nurses who have been assaulted report conflict between their roles as a professional and as a victim (Lanza 1985b). Nurses are not socialized to expect to be assault victims, and most do not receive any academic education to prepare them for such a fate. Any formal training usually comes through employment in a psychiatric facility. There are conflicting realities when a nurse is assaulted (Lanza 1985b). He or she generally believes that nurses are not assaulted, and yet it has occurred. There is also divided loyalty between allegiance to one's professional functioning (putting the patient's needs first) and attention to one's own needs as a victim (Lanza 1985b).

There are several examples of this dilemma. A nurse who is hit by a patient may be required to continue working because staffing is inadequate to permit him or her to go home. Family members question why their relative works in "such a place." The victim often defends the institution to family members and denies his or her own feelings of victimization. Nurses are in the somewhat unique position of needing to provide extensive care for a person who assaulted them. For example, the patient may require continuous observation by the nursing staff after assaulting one of the nursing staff members.

In summary, victims experience intense emotional reactions, want someone with whom to speak about their reactions, yet feel that it is "unprofessional" to do so. Victims do not expect to receive support from hospital administrators despite the victims' loyalty to the institution.

Interventions

The effort toward interventions is usually geared toward staff training in the early awareness and management of aggressive behavior. This is particularly important for risk management. Unfortunately, the effort often stops here perhaps because of the wish to believe that training will eliminate the problem of patients who assault. The reality is that although the risk of assault may be reduced, staff will continue to be assaulted, which is in part due to our poor prediction rate of assaultive behavior (Monahan 1981, 1989). Furthermore, a large percentage of patients do not give the usual clinical cues indicative of impending violence (Tanke and Yesavage 1985), and psychiatric hospitals now contain more seriously ill patients who are more prone to violence than in the past (Bachrack 1982; McCarrick and Manderscheid 1985; Miller and Maier 1987; Pepper and Rydiewicz 1981; Sosowsky 1980; Steadman et al. 1978).

There must be interventions that recognize the reality that staff are victimized and that assault is a serious job stressor (Browner 1987). A particularly useful intervention for staff who have been assaulted is to offer *supportive* counseling. *Supportive* is emphasized to indicate the importance of counseling that focuses on the victim's perceived needs and not those of hospital administrators. There is danger if the latter scenario exists that the victim will receive counseling "to improve his or her performance" and not to help the victim deal with his or her own unique reactions.

There are a variety of methods to offer counseling services to assault victims. The method is less crucial than is the importance of a supportive attitude. I now share the experience of one effective program.

Counseling Services

The formation of a victim assault support team (Lanza 1984b, 1985a) grew out of multidisciplinary concern with the plight of staff who had been assaulted. Until the inception of the support team, staff victims often sought support from coworkers. However, it was felt that a recognized service needed to be available for staff victims.

The development of the victim assault support team began as a grass-roots movement. Staff members from nursing, occupational therapy, psychiatry, psychology, and social work met to discuss the need for such a service as well as plans for implementation. The directors of the various services were contacted to provide input and support. The decision was made that the director would provide services initially. Based on an increase in the number of requests for victim support services, other counselors would be added to the team.

The qualifications for counselors were fairly broad as to formal academic preparation; however, one was expected to have training as a mental health professional. Beyond that, specific qualifications required that the counselor have an intimate acquaintance with the problem of patient assault. The counselor does not have to have had the experience of being an assault victim but does need the capacity to empathize with the victim. Although understanding the assault situation from the victim's perspective is essential, it is necessary not "to take the victim's side." The counselor must be objective to be able to provide support and guidance for the victim. For example, victims are often angry at administration for the assault. The counselor must be able to help the victim deal with the reality of those issues as well as any symbolic significance related to other areas in the victim's life.

It was decided that the services of the victim assault support team would be available to the victims at their request. Other staff members could suggest the use of the support services, but there is no requirement to do so. This was to protect the victim's wish for privacy and to provide freedom from unwanted pressure to seek counseling.

Because victim assault support services were only available to the victim at his or her request, it was necessary to publicize their existence widely. Advertisements in the form of announcements at various staff meetings, explanations of the service during educational programs, and notices in the hospital newspaper were made. The personnel health physician was also contacted because he or she generally examined the victim after an assault.

Most staff who sought counseling did so 1 week after being assaulted. Following the assault, victims reported feeling upset but then feeling better. They sought counseling after experiencing unexpected episodes of fearfulness and crying. Victims were distressed by these symptoms because they thought that they had coped with their feelings. Other reactions reported by victims were feeling anger at the patient, criticized and not supported by coworkers, humiliated, fearful of returning to work, stressed in having to cope with their families' concerns and with pressures to leave work, and anger at the amount of paperwork required to report the assault.

Victims were generally seen for two interviews. During the first interview, they reviewed symptoms that they experienced. The victims were helped to ventilate and understand the significance of their symptoms as part of what most victims experienced following an assault. The counselor provided anticipatory guidance about any additional reactions that might be experienced. In addition, specific coping strategies were explored, such as how to deal with the fear of returning to work.

Facilitating the victim's return to work was often accomplished by counselor-led meetings between the victim and staff and victim and assailant. The victim and staff meet to review the assault episode. There is exploration about how each person felt at the time of the assault and afterward. Issues of support for all as well as preventive measures are discussed. Coworkers often feel guilty about the assault regardless of the surrounding circumstances. The victim often experiences underlying anger toward coworkers and feels unsupported by them.

Meetings between the victim and assailant are important because both parties generally continue to interact on the same unit. Both explore their feelings about the assault and discuss parameters of their future relationship. Understanding what precipitated the assault and that violence will not be tolerated are essential outcomes (Felthous 1984).

Victims were encouraged to deal with family concerns by having open discussions with family members about family members' fears, sense of responsibility in wanting to protect the victim, and sometimes sense of guilt that the victim had been assaulted.

Usually a second appointment was made with the counselor 1 week later. Symptoms and coping strategies were again reviewed.

A useful instrument to assist in the counseling of assault victims is the Assault Response Questionnaire (Lanza 1988a). Measures of the intensity of victim reaction can be made as well as specific areas of stress identified. Reliability and validity properties are described.

Coping Strategies

The work of Janoff-Bulman and Frieze (1983) is particularly useful in its application to counseling assault victims. These authors detailed how three assumptions, which are shared by most people, are affected as a result of any victimization, regardless of the cause.

1. *The belief in personal invulnerability.* After victimization, the person is preoccupied with fear of reoccurrence. Prior to victimization, the "illusion of invulnerability" protects us from stress and anxiety.
2. *The perception of the world as meaningful and comprehensible.* One way for us to make sense of our world is to believe that it is controllable; for example, we can prevent misfortune by engaging in sufficiently cautious behaviors. The world does not appear meaningful to victims who feel they were cautious and are good people. The problem of loss of meaning focuses not on the question "Why did this event happen?" but rather on the question "Why did this event happen to me?" It is the selective incidence of victimization that appears to warrant explanation.
3. *The view of ourselves in a positive light.* The trauma activates negative self-images. Many victims see themselves as weak, helpless, needy, frightened, and out of control. They may also experience a sense of deviance. They feel as if they were "singled out for misfortune" and that this sets them off as different from other people.

Coping involves coming to terms with shattered assumptions—coming to terms with a world in which bad things can and do happen to oneself. Although the victim is not apt to ever view himself or herself again as entirely invulnerable, the victim will still need to work on establishing a view of the world as not wholly malevolent or threatening.

The assumptions of vulnerability, meaning, and self-esteem will be examined, altered, and reexamined until one's victimization and conceptual system are consistent.

Redefining the victimization. The victim may selectively evaluate his or her victimization by comparing with less fortunate others, comparing on a basis of favorable attitude, creating hypothetical worse worlds, construing benefit from the experience, and manufacturing normative standards of adjustment. How one evaluates the victimization affects the extent to which the victimization functions as a stressor and threat.

Making sense of the event. One way of making sense of an event is to find some purpose in it. If the victimization can be viewed as serving a purpose, the victim is able to reestablish a belief in an orderly, comprehensible world.

Blaming oneself is one way of explaining why the event occurred to oneself in particular. Self-blame can be functional, particularly if it involves attributions to one's behavior rather than to enduring personality characteristics. Behavioral self-blame allows attributions to a controllable and modifiable source. Victims can alter their behavior. Thus the victim believes he or she can avoid being victimized in the future. Characterological attributions are associated with depression. Behavioral responses are not helpful for victims who felt that they engaged in safe or in cautious practices prior to their victimization. Rules that had provided them with a personal sense of invulnerability did not work, and their perception of safety and security was destroyed. Those who feel most invulnerable prior to victimization may have the most difficulty in coping after victimization.

The Role of Administrators

There is a prevailing stereotype that administrators are uncaring about nurses who are assaulted (Lanza 1983, 1984a). However, those in administrative positions did not see themselves as insensitive to staff who had been assaulted or as engaging in blaming behaviors (Lanza 1988c).

If the latter view has validity, one may wonder why nursing administrators have not been more public in their recognition of patient assault as a problem facing nursing. For example, very little appeared in the nursing literature before the late 1980s about reactions to caring for the assaultive patient or the frequency of patient assault (Lanza 1983). Two possibilities exist to explain this lack of recognition. The first is that nurses in high-level positions may have had few or no experiences of being assaulted by a patient and are thus not aware that the problem exists. A significant inverse correlation was found between level of job and experience with patient assault ($r = -.18$, $P < .05$) (Lanza 1988c). The second possibility is that nurses in high-level positions may not see themselves as potential assault victims. Nurses with high-level positions saw themselves as influencing their own environment rather than being victims of fate and tended to avoid rather than acknowledge their own stressful reactions (Lanza 1988c).

One may ask if administrators should not be more public in their acknowledgment that patient assault is a problem. On closer inspection, there may be conflict for administrators in doing so. If administrators admit that patient assault is a problem at their institution, the administrators may find themselves blamed for the problem. For example, the assumption could be made that patient assault is a problem because of poor administration. It could also be suggested that if the patients become violent, it is because they are mistreated. In fact, as earlier mentioned, issues of patients' rights and safety measures to prevent violence are often presented as adversarial. When institution of safety measures is being considered, patients' rights are seen to be at risk rather than the more global approach being taken—that only when safety exists can anyone (staff or patients) have rights. The last dilemma to be faced in publicizing the existence of patient assaultiveness is that such knowledge may arouse fear in the community and inhibit the discharge of nonviolent patients. All patients with a history of mental illness may then be seen as too dangerous to live outside of the hospital—a long-held belief that mental health professionals have valiantly tried to eradicate.

Given that coming to terms with the problem of patient assault may arouse ambivalent feelings and conflict-laden situations, there are steps that administrators can take to support nursing staff in dealing with the assaultive situation:

1. Support the legitimation of patient assault as a frequent problem with which nursing staff must deal. Publicity can be achieved through meetings, journal articles, and the media.
2. Support nursing staff assault victims through direct administrative contact as well as nonjudgmental, supportive counseling to help victims cope with their reactions.
3. Confront the myth of blaming the victim for the assault. Too often the nurse-victim is blamed for the assault regardless of the circumstances; for example, "She used poor judgment" or "He pushed the patient too far." A nurse may have used poor judgment, but this does not justify that the nurse was assaulted.
4. Establish an alliance with nursing staff in an investigation of the problem of patient assault at one's institution. In a collaborative fashion, develop programs to cope with and prevent violence.

5. Encourage research on different aspects of patient assault in nursing practice. Patient violence is an important and long-standing issue that is only beginning to be studied.

Future Directions

Approaching the problem of assaultive behavior from a holistic perspective is essential if the problem is to be adequately addressed. Using Monahan's (1981, 1989) framework to examine the interaction of the assailant, others involved, and the environment is important. Major efforts have been directed to understanding the assaultive patient. Most of the focus on the others or staff has been aimed at training for preventing assaults. That staff are victimized is the neglected element that has much potential impact on the problem of assault. Their plight is not realistically addressed. They are told to perform better. A useful approach is to examine the interaction of participants in assault (Lanza and Kayne, unpublished report, 1990). Intra- and interpsychodynamic issues of patients and staff involved in an assault can be explored using a qualitative approach. A methodology such as grounded theory (Glaser and Strauss 1967) would yield rich and in-depth data.

In a time of austerity measures and budget cuts, adequate staffing and support services to staff are often among the first to go. "Do more with less" is the common refrain. Those making such decisions often are unaware that staffing levels are related to numbers of assaults (Lanza et al. 1992), the outcomes of assaults, and the fact that assaults are so vastly underreported. In fact, much important information about assault is confined to a fairly closed system at the staff level. This may be due to bureaucratic inefficiency or, more likely, staff alienation from higher management. Whatever the reason, wise administrators who are concerned with clinical issues will insist on realistically safe staffing levels and adequate resources. To do less will diminish the likelihood of therapeutic milieu-based programs and encourage prisonlike atmospheres in our mental health settings.

References

Adler W, Kresger C, Ziegler P: Patient violence in a private psychiatric hospital, in Assault Within Psychiatric Facilities. Edited by Lion JR, Reid WH. New York, Grune & Stratton, 1983, pp 81–89

Bachrack L: Young adult chronic patients: an analytic review of the literature. Hosp Community Psychiatry 22:189–198, 1982

Bernstein HA: Survey of threats and assaults directed towards psychotherapists. Am J Psychother 35:542–549, 1981

Binder RL, McNeil DE: Victims and families of violent psychiatric patients. Bull Am Acad Psychiatry Law 14:131–139, 1986

Brizer DA, Crowner ML, Convit A, et al: Clinical and research report. Am J Psychiatry 145:751–752, 1988

Browner CH: Job stress and health: the role of social support at work. Res Nurs Health 10:93–100, 1987

Carmel H, Hunter M: Staff injuries from inpatient violence. Hosp Community Psychiatry 40:41–46, 1989

Colson DB, Allen JG, Coyne L, et al: Patterns of staff perception of difficult patients in a long-term psychiatric hospital. Hosp Community Psychiatry 36:168–172, 1985

Colson DB, Allen JG, Coyne L, et al: Profiles of difficult psychiatric hospital patients. Hosp Community Psychiatry 37:720–724, 1986

Conn LM, Lion JR: Assault in a university hospital, in Assault Within Psychiatric Facilities. Edited by Lion JR, Reid WH. New York, Grune & Stratton, 1983, pp 61–69

Cust K: Assault: just part of the job? Canadian Nurse 82:19–20, 1986

Drinkwater JM: Violence in Psychiatric Hospitals: Development in the Study of Criminal Behavior, Vol 2. London, Academic Press, 1982

Felthous AR: Preventing assaults on a psychiatric ward. Hosp Community Psychiatry 35:1223–1226, 1984

Glaser BG, Strauss AL: Discovery of Grounded Theory: Strategies for Qualitative Research. Chicago, IL, Aldine, 1967

Halleck S: Legal and ethical acts of behavior control, in Biomedical Ethics. Edited by Mappes TA, Zembaty JS. New York, McGraw-Hill, 1974, pp 267–273

Hodgkinson PE, McIvor L, Phillips M: Patient assaults on staff in a psychiatric hospital: a two year retrospective study. Med Sci Law 25:288–294, 1985

Ionno JA: A prospective study on assaultive behavior in female psychiatric patients, in Assault Within Psychiatric Facilities. Edited by Lion JR, Reid WH. New York, Grune & Stratton, 1983, pp 71–80

Janoff-Bulman R, Frieze IH: A theoretical perspective for understanding reactions to victimization. Journal of Social Issues 39:1–17, 1983

Lanza ML: Violence by patients is a complex problem (letter). Boston Globe, August 1, 1982

Lanza ML: The reactions of nursing staff to physical assault by a patient. Hosp Community Psychiatry 34:44–47, 1983

Lanza ML: Factors affecting blame placement for assault upon nurses. Issues in Mental Health Nursing 6:143–162, 1984a

Lanza ML: Victim assault support team for staff. Hosp Community Psychiatry 35:414, 1984b

Lanza ML: Counseling services for staff victims of patient assault. Administration in Mental Health Services 12:205–207, 1985a

Lanza ML: How do nurses react to patient assault? J Psychosoc Nurs Ment Health Serv 23:6–11, 1985b

Lanza ML: Relationship of severity of assault to blame placement for assault. Arch Psychiatr Nurs 1:269–279, 1987

Lanza ML: Assault Response Questionnaire. Issues in Mental Health Nursing 9:17–29, 1988a

Lanza ML: Factors relevant to patient assault. Issues in Mental Health Nursing 9:239–258, 1988b

Lanza ML: Reactions of nurses to a patient assault vignette. West J Nurs Res 10:45–54, 1988c

Lanza ML: Blaming the victim: complex (non-linear) patterns of counsel attributions by nurses in response to vignettes vignettes of a patient assaulting a nurse. Journal of Emergency Nursing 17:229–309, 1991

Lanza ML, Kayne H, Hicks C, et al: Patient assault: a comparison of staff and patient perceptions. Paper presented at the Nursing Research Network of Boston Annual Conference, Boston, MA, New England Deaconess Hospital, June 2, 1992

Lehmann LS, Padilla M, Clark S, et al: Training personnel in the prevention and management of violent behavior. Hosp Community Psychiatry 34:40–43, 1983

Lion JR, Snyder W, Merrill G: Underreporting of assaults on staff in a state hospital. Hosp Community Psychiatry 32:497–498, 1981

Mappes J, Zembaty J (eds): Biomedical Ethics. New York, McGraw-Hill, 1981

McCarrick A, Manderscheid R: Correlate of acting out among young adult chronic patients. Hosp Community Psychiatry 8:847–852, 1985

Miller RD, Maier G: Factors affecting the decision to prosecute mental patients for criminal behavior. Hosp Community Psychiatry 38:50–55, 1987

Monahan J: The Clinical Prediction of Violent Behavior. Washington DC, US Department of Health and Human Services, 1981

Monahan J: Predicting violence among the mentally ill. Audio Digest—Psychiatry Vol 18, Tape 21, 1989

Pearson M, Wilmot E, Padi M: A study of violent behavior among in-patients in a psychiatric hospital. Br J Psychiatry 142:232–235, 1986

Pepper B, Rydiewicz H: The young adult chronic patient: overview of a population. Hosp Community Psychiatry 32:463–469, 1981

Reid WH, Bolligner MF, Edwards G: Assaults in hospitals. Bull Am Acad Psychiatry Law 13:1–4, 1985

Rix G: Staff sickness and its relationship to violent incidents on a regional secure psychiatric unit. J Adv Nurs 12:223–228, 1987

Ryan W: Blaming the Victim. New York, Vintage, 1976

Scalfani M: Violence and behavior control. J Psychosoc Nurs Ment Health Serv 24:8–13, 1986

Silver JM, Yudofsky SC: Documentation of aggression in the assessment of the violent patient. Psychiatric Annals 17:375–384, 1987

Soloff PH: Emergency management of violent patients, in Psychiatry Update: American Psychiatric Association Annual Review, Vol 6. Edited by Hales RE, Frances AJ. Washington, DC, American Psychiatric Press, 1987, pp 510–536

Sosowsky L: Number of patient violence. Arch Psychiatr Nurs 1:280–284, 1980

Steadman HJ, Cocozza JJ, Melick ME: Explaining the increased arrest rate among mental patients: the changing clientele of state hospitals. Am J Psychiatry 137:1602–1605, 1978

Tanke ED, Yesavage JA: Characteristics of assaultive patients who do and do not provide visible cues of potential violence. Am J Psychiatry 142:1409–1413, 1985

Tardiff K: Characteristics of assaultive patients in private hospitals. Am J Psychiatry 141:1234–1235, 1984

Tardiff K, Koenigsberg HW: Assaultive behavior among psychiatric outpatients. Am J Psychiatry 142:960–963, 1985

Ulrich L: Mental illness and the dilemma of behavioral control, in Biomedical Ethics. Edited by Mappes TA, Zembaty JS. New York, McGraw-Hill, 1978, pp 280–286

Wortman C: Causal attributions and personal control, in New Directions in Attribution Research, Vol 1. Edited by Harvey JH. New York, Wiley, 1976, pp 23–52

Chapter 9

A Critical Incident Report for Capturing Violent Acts: The North Carolina Experience

David B. Langmeyer, Ph.D.

To develop a realistic awareness of violence toward clinicians, an institution must have some reliable mechanism for assessing the amount of violence. Such an assessment tool must be reliable and valid. Without such a tool, hospital violence as gauged, for example, by the usual nursing incident method has been estimated to underreport assaultive behavior by a factor of five (Lion et al. 1981). Moreover, if assaultive behavior is only cataloged through standard nursing reports, it tends to become "lost" in the midst of other elements of the reports, such as patient falls, medication errors, and patient elopements. Often, nursing incident reports are not computerized so that comparison rates over time, or comparative aspects of a particular type of incident, cannot be determined without tedious review by hand.

In this chapter, I report an alternative mechanism for recording assaultive behavior developed by the Division of Mental Health for the state of North Carolina beginning in 1986. An incident report form was developed with simple but consistent definitions of assaultive behavior and of injury. The report mechanism was implemented within all four state psychiatric hospitals following staff training, and it was housed

This project was completed in collaboration with the psychiatric hospital quality assurance coordinators L. Jolliff, S. Wilkes, M. Sudderth, and J. Southerland. The systems analysis and programming to produce and automate the patient incident form was done by T. Wildfire.

within the quality assurance program of the hospitals.

The report documented the frequency, location, patient(s), and severity of assaults. It also provided information concerning time of day and staffing ratios at the time of assault. dBASE programming was used to prepare graphic and tabular summaries of the data; the summaries were utilized at both the state level (for interhospital comparisons and interventions) and at the hospital level (for unit and patient comparisons and local interventions). This tool has been readily accepted and used by the North Carolina mental health system. It provides a solid database for critical policy decisions such as staffing ratios and the identification and "special handling" of highly assaultive patients. The following is the history of its inception.

Background

In the summer of 1986, the issue of violence within North Carolina state psychiatric hospitals became politically prominent. An ad hoc committee, comprising primarily physicians from each of the four state psychiatric hospitals but also including representation by the hospitals' quality assurance coordinators, and the state Director of the Division of Mental Health met to formulate a concrete response to this issue. One of the first problems the group faced was the lack of consistent, reliable, and believable information about the amount and consequences of violence in the state psychiatric institutions. Although a time-limited study had been conducted in 1984, nothing more recent was available to the task force. Because each of the state hospitals had its own methods of collecting information, varying definitions of *violence* were used. Although anecdotal impressions as to the extent of violence abounded, no one knew how much violence, in reality, was occurring.

In 3 short months, the task force implemented a systematic, standardized data-gathering system that the local hospitals approved. This success is attributed to a few early decisions and approaches. Despite the state Office of Mental Health's needing these data critically and on a timely basis, the focus of the task force was not presented as a top-down demand. Rather, the effort was constructed as a hospital-driven system. The primary use of the information was for *hospital* management, with summary information needed periodically at the state level. Thus, the procedures developed were flexible and broad enough to meet the individualized needs of the multiple hospitals.

A second strategy was that the data collection methods had to recognize who was actually filling out the incident forms, how the forms were to be transmitted to the quality assurance office, and how the quality assurance office was going to maintain the data. Usually, the recorders were the mental health technicians who might only have a high school level of formal education and who had multiple tasks to complete on busy wards during their shifts. Without a well-rehearsed procedure for data transfer with identified responsible staff accountable for the transfer, data would be lost. Also, without a user-friendly data entry and retrieval system, quality assurance and hospital administration would never have the data in a form from which to generate reasonable policy.

Third, the task force based its strategy on the technology of small, inexpensive microcomputers to handle the large quantities of data that could still utilize sophisticated database and statistical software. Consequently, data storage and analysis could be programmed in familiar programs and run locally on locally maintained and controlled microcomputers rather than being maintained on mainframe computers in the central mental health office.

Development of the Reporting System

The task force was given a deadline for completion of the project (January 1, 1987). The task force was empowered to call on resources within each of the hospitals; the director of the Division of Mental Health at times intervened to ensure that resources were made available by the four hospital directors for programming, data entry, and other project needs. Thus, the high priority of this project was tangibly communicated to the hospital directors.

In addition to strong administrative support, the composition of the development group was critical. There was a central representative for each psychiatric hospital, namely, the existing quality assurance coordinator who already was collecting data and reporting on violence. One person from the state central office was a permanent member of the group functioning primarily in a technical capacity; another central office staff member did the computer programming. The administrative message was clear: This was to be a predominantly hospital-based effort.

The reporting of violence had been disjointed and ad hoc. Within the four hospital systems, various reporting mechanisms were already in place: "24-hour report," special reports for drug reactions, reports for medical "code blues," reports cataloging restraint and seclusion, and reports for self-inflicted injuries. The standardization of violence reporting became an opportunity to consolidate much of the other incident reporting and to reduce the burden on ward nurses and health care technicians. Through consolidation, the violence reporting effort led to the creation of the patient incident form (Figure 9–1). A simplification of reporting procedures within the hospitals helped it to gain acceptance by the clinical staff.

The state office had the most interest in the type of violence that either did or could result in injury as noted in the incident form specifications. Physical assaults were only one kind of violence that occurred on the hospital units. Verbal aggressive behavior was also significant and contributed to the perception that there was an unsafe situation. Nevertheless, in the development of the North Carolina patient incident form, it was decided that verbal aggressive behavior would not be captured in this report. The task force felt that the labeling of verbal behavior as aggressive often was unrelated to the behavior itself and would be quite difficult to standardize across staff, wards, and hospitals. For example, the task force felt that experienced staff who were dealing with known patients would tolerate verbal behavior that was louder and went on longer than would a new staff member dealing with unfamiliar patients. This would lead to variability in the threshold for reporting such behavior as "an incident" and could lead to lower levels of verbal aggressive behavior being reported at hospitals with more experienced staff and lower patient turnover rates. In contrast, physical assaults were readily accepted as being more reliably reportable and also were the target of interest for both the state and hospital management.

In keeping with the principle that the methods and the information should be tailored for the optimal use of each hospital, data elements were developed so that a core of items would be common for all of the four hospitals, but individual hospitals could include additional codes for their own use. This permitted comparability across hospitals for items that were of interest to the state but still let the hospitals include items that were of local interest. For example, medical items such as "code blue" or "diabetic coma" were included in some but not all of the

USE BALL POINT PEN
PRESS DOWN HARD

PATIENT INCIDENT/OCCURENCE REPORT
(See instructions on back)

Date of incident:______________ Time of incident:__________ HB 95: ___YES ___NO

Ward/bldg:______________ Attending physician:____________________________

Number staff present where incident occurred:_________

Census:_________ Number staff with minor injury_________ Number staff with major injury_________

[NOTE: EMPLOYEE INJURY REPORT MUST BE COMPLETED ON EACH INJURED EMPLOYEE] (ADDRESSOGRAPH)

TYPE OF INCIDENT

SECTION I

ASSAULTS

A__Attack on property
B__Attack on other not resulting in injury to victim
C__Attack on other resulting in minor injury to victim
D__Attack on other resulting in major injury to victim
E__Attack on other resulting in death
F__Fire setting
G__Sexual attack on other

OTHER

B__Victim of sexual assault
C__Choking
I__Victim of physical assault
J__Self-injurious behavior
K__Suicide
L__Suicide attempt
M__Fall
N__Accident other than fall
O__Injury of unknown origin
R__Unusual death (other than suicide)
S__Risk management
T__Other____________

NOTE: IS THIS A SERIOUS INCIDENT ACCORDING TO DEFINITION ON BACK OF THIS FORM? ___NO ___YES

SECTION II

SEVERITY OF INJURY OR DAMAGE

Injury to this patient
A__None
B__Minor
C__Major
D__Death

Property Damage
A__None
B__Less than $50.00
C__More than $50.00

LOCATION

B__Bedroom
C__Bathroom
D__Dayroom
E__On ward hall
F__Elevator
G__Stairway
H__Clinic
I__Grounds
L__Dining room
M__Activity area
N__Off ward hall
O__Unknown
P__Other__________

INVOLVEMENT

A__Patient only
B__Patient/patient
C__Patient/staff
D__Patient/patient/staff
E__Patient/visitor
F__Other__________

KEY: Minor injury: bruises, sprains, welts, etc., requiring first aid or less
Major injury: broken bones, lacerations requiring sutures, internal injury, etc., requiring more than first aid

SECTION III

WITNESS: ____________________________

ACCOUNT OF EVENT: ____________________________

SECTION IV

PATIENT INTERVENTION REQUIRED

B__Talked to patient
C__Time-out/quiet room
D__Close observation
E__One/one observation
F__Suicidal precautions
G__Holding patient/PIT
H__Restraint
I__Seclusion
J__Restraint and seclusion
K__Immediate medication by mouth
L__Immediate medication by injection
M__Immediate medical or nursing treatment
N__CPR
O__Heimlich maneuver
P__Other__________

Signature/Title:______________________ Date:__________ Time:__________

SECTION V

PHYSICIAN REPORT (If medical care was necessary)____________________________

Physician signature:______________________ Date:__________ Time:__________

DISTRIBUTION: Within 48 hrs, original and 1st copy to Standards Management Director; 2nd copy to Nursing Manager/Program Director

DDH 11-116-89 (Rev. 8/89)

Figure 9–1. Patient incident form.

hospital forms in response to quality assurance concerns of medical staff. Thus, flexibility and local "ownership" were achieved while comparability was maintained for shared items. Technically, the information on the form was coded and entered using dBASE III+.[1]

After the hospitals had used the original reporting form for a pilot year, minor changes were made following regular reports back to the task force about how the form was being used, as well as accepted, by the ward staff. A major revision was not deemed advisable because the ward staff would have needed retraining and the reprogramming costs would have been prohibitive. However, some coding changes were made, and a clarification of the cataloging and reporting of staff injuries was accomplished. This revision process seemed to strengthen the feeling of the various hospital staff that this was, indeed, *their* form. They felt "listened to," and a form modification had resulted from their request.

The Patient Incident Form

The patient incident form that is currently in use (Figure 9–1) includes sections that are captured on an automated database: the type of incident, the severity of injury or damage, the location of the incident within the hospital, the involvement of other people, and the type of interventions that were required as a result of the incident. Information is also captured that includes the time and date of the incident, whether the person was on a court order for violent criminal behavior (North Carolina "House Bill 95" patients), the attending physician, the number of staff actually present at the time, the census on the ward that day, and the number of staff who received injury from the incident.

A form is completed on each patient who is involved. The patient who initiated the assault is coded for "assaults," and any other patient involved is coded as "victim of physical assault" in the "other" cate-

---

[1]It permitted simple reports to be prepared in dBASE. Most of the reports were intended to be run from a menu so that the staff in the quality assurance section of the hospital would not have to become proficient in dBASE. dBASE also allowed the records to be prepared for output in a standard data format (ASCII code with line feed and carriage return after each record), which could serve as input to other more sophisticated statistical programs that run on microcomputers.

gory. All forms related to one incident are kept together so that they are counted as one incident and given a consecutive code. Therefore, there is an individual record for each person involved as well as an "incident record" that can be generated from the incident number.

For consistency across hospitals, definitions are critical as well as reliability training for the recorders. *Minor injury* is defined as bruises, sprains, welts, and other injuries that require first aid or less and can be treated on the ward. *Major injury* involves broken bones, lacerations requiring sutures, internal injury, and other injuries that require more than first aid and treatment off the ward.

To simplify reporting and reduce the time required for reporting, the instructions for completing the incident report are printed on the back of each form. Consequently, the staff member filling out the form does not have to go to an instruction manual to complete the form (see Figure 9–2).

Each record is sent to the quality assurance office of the local hospital, where it is edited to make certain that it is completely filled out and that the information is internally consistent. The quality assurance staff is in regular contact with ward staff to clarify the characteristics of an incident when the form does not appear to be correct.

Analysis of the Data

The major categories under each section are captured independently of each other. This means that one code can be entered for assaults, significant drug reaction, other, injury to this patient only, property damage, location, and involvement and *three* codes entered for patient intervention required. This allows codes within each category to be counted and cross-tabulations to be calculated as well. For example, the number of various assaults can be produced as well as the location of the various assaults, or the time of day, or the unit and ward on which the assaults took place. Specific report examples are provided next.

Utilization of Reports: The State Level

The major interest for the state Office of Mental Health is the category of assaults and the victims of physical assaults. On a quarterly basis, each hospital's quality assurance coordinator sends to the state office

INSTRUCTIONS

GENERAL: Complete at time incident occurs.
Complete all blanks applying to this patient in this incident.
Document account of incident and treatment rendered, if any, in patient's chart in progress notes also, and report incident to patient's attending physician.

TOP SECTION: Complete all identifying information.
Indicate number staff present in area where incident initially occurred (not number staff on duty or elsewhere).
Census should be Daily Census on ward the day of the incident.
If any staff injured in this incident, indicate total number with minor and/or major injury. All staff injuries must also be reported on Employee Injury Form DDH 51-21-87.

SECTION I: TYPE OF INCIDENT
Assaults—Complete this column only on the patient initiating a violent act. Complete a separate form on each patient victim of this assault and attach all forms together so the incident will be counted as one incident. If the incident is mutual aggression or if the patient initiating the assault is unknown, complete a separate form on each patient indicating each as the attacker and clip forms together.

SECTION II: SEVERITY OF INJURY/DAMAGE
Patient Injury—Indicate severity of injury suffered by patient on whom this incident report is being filed.
Property Damage—Complete only if the incident involved property and/or objects.
LOCATION—Complete this section for all incidents.
INVOLVEMENT—Complete for all incidents. Check "C" or "D" only when staff was intentionally attacked, accidently injured in the process of intervening, or if patient was accidently injured by staff. Routine involvement by staff is reported in Section IV.

SECTION III: Give name(s) of witness(es) if applicable and describe what happened in this incident. If more space is needed, complete on blank sheet and attach to form. If assault, indicate names of all patients involved and attach separate incident report forms on each patient.

SECTION IV: PATIENT INTERVENTION REQUIRED
Complete on all incidents.
You may check up to three interventions; if more were used, check the three most restrictive/intrusive and use blank lines under "other" to indicate additional interventions.
Sign name and title of person preparing report; indicate date and time.

SECTION V: PHYSICIAN REPORT—To be completed by physician only if medical care was required.

DEFINITION: SERIOUS INCIDENT

SERIOUS INCIDENTS are assaults involving weapons or resulting in major injury; self-injurious behavior resulting in major injury; serious suicide attempts; nonconsenting sexual activity; unusual death; or any other event which in staff judgment has substantive impact on the patient or the unit and/or has potential risk management implications for the hospital.

Serious incidents shall also be reported on the 24-hour report, including names of patients involved. If incident is unusual death or nonconsenting sexual activity, staff shall immediately notify by phone the Hospital Director (or Administrative Physician on-call after hours).

Figure 9–2. Instructions for the patient incident form.

the data for that quarter.[2] The data are reviewed at the state level, and a file is created that contains the reports of assaults and victims of assault. From this file, reports are generated for each hospital that count the number and type of assaults and report on the extent of injury to patients and staff resulting from physical assaults and fire setting.

Table 9–1 is an illustration of the quarterly report form, the last quarter of 1989, for the North Carolina state psychiatric hospital system. The number of various types of assault is listed for each hospital. This type of table, generated at the state level, is produced using a statistical analysis program (BASS) and is slightly edited to make the program more readable. The output from the statistical program can be modified using most word-processing packages. Without the editing, the legends for the hospitals and the types of assault would be one-letter codes. It is highly recommended that reports be presented with recognizable labels rather than raw data codes.

Table 9–2 and Table 9–3 report the number of patients and staff who were hurt as a result of violent acts. These tables separate minor and major injury. Because the hospitals are all different in size, differences in the number of assaults or injuries may be due to the size of the hospital or patient census. To take size into account and make comparisons easier, another report (see Table 9–4) is generated that calculates the frequency of assault and injury for the resident population for a particular time period (the number of assaults per 100 residents over the quarter of reporting), allowing cross-hospital comparisons as well as cross-year comparisons.

Utilization of Reports: The Hospital Level

Greatest interest at the individual hospitals has been on the *trends* in violence—time comparisons by month, quarter, and year—as well as on the performance of individual units and wards. Depending on the capabilities available to the quality assurance coordinators, presentation of this information ranges from simple frequency tables to two-way tables or graphs.

---

[2]The data are sent by diskette. The generation of the diskette is automated and can be run from a menu where the beginning and ending dates are specified.

Table 9–1. Number of violent incidents, including severity of outcome, fourth quarter, 1989

	Hospital				
Incident	**Broughton**	**Cherry**	**Dix**	**Umstead**	**Total**
Attack on property					
N	17	44	54	15	130
Row %	13.08	33.85	41.54	11.54	
Column %	8.67	11.76	13.88	5.64	10.61
Attack with no injury					
N	70	146	212	136	564
Row %	12.41	25.89	37.59	24.11	
Column %	35.71	39.04	54.50	51.13	46.04
Attack with minor injury					
N	100	168	120	107	495
Row %	20.20	33.94	24.24	21.62	
Column %	51.02	44.92	30.85	40.23	40.41
Attack with major injury					
N	7	15	1	5	28
Row %	25.00	53.57	3.57	17.86	
Column %	3.57	4.01	0.26	1.88	2.29
Fire setting					
N	1	0	0	3	4
Row %	25.00	0	0	75.00	
Column %	0.51	0	0	1.13	0.33
Sexual attack					
N	1	1	2	0	4
Row %	25.00	25.00	50.00	0	
Column %	0.51	0.27	0.51	0	0.33
Total					
N	196	374	389	266	1,225
Row %	16.00	30.53	31.76	21.71	100.00

Each hospital is provided with the capability of running a summary report from a menu. This report summarizes the information contained on the patient incident form for the hospital as a whole and for each unit in the hospital. There is also a ward report that lists the individual incidents and an abbreviated summary. This final report allows the ward staff to validate the information that was recorded during the past month.

Table 9–2. Number of patients injured as a result of violence, fourth quarter, 1989

Incident	Hospital				
	Broughton	**Cherry**	**Dix**	**Umstead**	**Total**
Minor injury					
N	153	185	107	120	565
Row %	27.08	32.74	18.94	21.24	
Column %	89.47	91.13	94.69	97.56	92.62
Major injury					
N	18	18	6	3	45
Row %	40.00	40.00	13.33	6.67	
Column %	10.53	8.87	5.31	2.44	7.38
Total					
N	171	203	113	123	610
Row %	28.03	33.28	18.52	20.16	100.00

Table 9–3. Number of staff injured as a result of patient violence, fourth quarter, 1989

Hospital	Minor injury	Major injury
Broughton	34	0
Cherry	21	2
Dix	79	1
Umstead	19	3

The summary report is made simple to read. Codes are written out in full so that one can read the report without referring to a code guide. The report is a simple frequency of incident report, with totals listed for 1) the number of reports entered, 2) the number of discrete incidents, 3) sex, 4) marital status, 5) race, 6) the number of staff with various levels of injury, 7) the average staffing per report, 8) the average daily census, 9) the number of reports for each day of the week, 10) the number of reports for each shift, 11) the frequency of each type of assault, 12) the frequency of each type of drug reaction, 13) the frequency of each type of "other" response, 14) the number of patient injuries by level of injury, 15) the frequency of property damage, 16) the number of reports for each location, 17) the number of reports

Table 9–4. Rates for various measures of hospital violence, fourth quarter, 1989 (rate per 100 resident population)

	Hospital			
Measures	**Broughton**	**Cherry**	**Dix**	**Umstead**
Incident				
Property	2.09	5.75	9.06	2.23
Others, no injury	8.62	19.08	35.57	20.18
Others, minor injury	12.32	21.96	20.13	15.88
Others, major injury	.86	1.96	.17	.74
Fire setting	.12	0	0	.45
Severity of patient injury				
Minor	18.84	24.18	17.95	17.80
Major	2.22	2.35	1.01	.45
Severity of staff injury				
Minor	4.19	2.75	13.26	2.82
Major	0	.26	.17	.45

for each type of involvement, and 18) the frequency of interventions required. This report is generated for the hospital as a whole and for each unit.

Most of the hospitals combine the individual unit reports into a hospital-wide report presented by unit for comparison. This is done manually at two of the hospitals and is done using BASS at the other two.[3]

The data can also be presented graphically. A bar graph showing the frequency of reports for each shift illustrates immediately when most of the incidents take place. A bar graph for each day of the week serves the same purpose. Graphs by unit allow clinical monitoring of units having a concentration of violent acts.

---

[3]The statistical package has been simplified by writing the report commands as a utility report in batch mode. The program can then be run from a menu rather than by having to know anything about the statistical program. At this time, the output is not labeled, so it cannot be easily read without a coding guide. However, it does give unit comparison information to the quality assurance coordinators without it having to be compiled manually.

The reports and information from these reports are clearly used at each hospital. However, the governance structure is different for each hospital, so it is not possible succinctly to report as to which committees review this information. Critical review, however, is done through a mechanism of thresholds. Each hospital has set a threshold level for violent acts based on a 2-year preceding history. If that threshold is exceeded, administrative and clinical reviews are initiated to determine what is happening on the outlier unit and to take corrective action. Critical individual incidents, flagged by this system, also may prompt administrative and clinical review. Information from these reports becomes a permanent part of the quality assurance committee's agenda and has received commendations from the Joint Commission on Accreditation of Healthcare Organizations' reviews.

Illustrative Results

At the inception of the centralized reporting project, anecdotal reports had suggested that there was an epidemic of significant violence within North Carolina state psychiatric hospitals. However, the occurrence of violent acts that resulted in major injury to patients or staff was demonstrated to be lower than anticipated. During the last quarter of 1989, for example, 6 staff in four hospitals had reported major injury, and 45 patients had reported major injury. The rate of major injury for patients was not equal across the hospitals, a finding that prompted attention to be focused on the hospitals and units where major injury occurred.

Although focusing the examination of assaults in relation to days of the week and shifts provided interesting findings, it varied for each hospital and did not illustrate a systemwide finding. In contrast, examination of the individuals who assaulted demonstrated that 50% of the assaultive incidents were committed by less than 15% of those who engaged in a violent act. To describe this differently, approximately 5% of the hospitals' resident population accounted for 50% of the assaultive acts. Such an observation clearly raises the possibility of targeted interventions for this portion of the hospital population.

Conclusions

In this chapter, I have described the successful implementation of a statewide recording system to record the number and characteristics of assaultive behavior within the state of North Carolina's psychiatric hospital system. Such a system abolishes the denial that assaults occur within such a system but demonstrates their characteristics devoid of anecdote or the potential for political distortion. Once standardized, such a system allows for interward and interhospital comparisons to improve management strategies by flagging those programs that are most successful at violence reduction. Similarly, comparisons over time can be made to correlate hospital violence with resource allocation, changes in state commitment laws, or internal hospital management policies. The development of such a standard database becomes the foundation for violence reduction and concomitantly enhanced clinician safety.

Reference

Lion JR, Snyder W, Merrill GL: Underreporting of assaults on staff in a state hospital. Hosp Community Psychiatry 32:497–498, 1981

Chapter 10

Strategies for Clinician Safety

Burr S. Eichelman, M.D., Ph.D.

The authors of preceding chapters have addressed the reality of clinician assault within inpatient settings, as verbal assault, with weapons, and within the training period of the psychiatric residency. Although there is considerable work to be done to understand and predict patient violence, there are many concrete interventions currently available to clinicians that can substantially enhance clinician safety and minimize the untoward effects of assault when it does occur. These interventions can be made at many organizational levels: political, institutional, unit, and personal.

Political Strategies

Many of the interventions described in this chapter require the allocation of resources for implementation. Such resources may be required for the purchase of equipment or for architectural changes. They may be the allocation of increased staff positions for safer care or even for data collection.

In the present economic climate, few new resources will be forthcoming without a significant educational effort at the political level. An example of such an action can be seen within the North Carolina mental health system. In the mid-1980s, a patient's death by assault became a political catalyst for both an *internal* effort, led by the administrators and clinicians within the four-hospital division of mental health, and an

---

Products mentioned within this chapter are provided only as illustrations. Their citation does not indicate endorsement or recommendation.

external effort, led by the administrative staff of the North Carolina Alliance for the Mentally Ill, for the state legislators to create a Mental Health Study Commission charged with examining violence within the state mental health system. One outcome of this commission was the recommendation and successful appropriation of state monies for additional staff within the state hospital system.

To provide the political process with accurate data in its lobbying effort, the state's Division of Mental Health supported the development and implementation of a new and more sensitive system for reporting assaultive behavior. This has been described by Langmeyer (Chapter 9, this volume). In short, the state hospitals and their administrators adopted the position that accurate portrayal of the clinical reality of hospital assaults was required—despite the potential for short-term political embarrassment—to reach an awareness of the problem at the legislative level to receive enhanced resources.

Not all hospital systems are this forward looking. W. H. Reid and associates (1985) noted that many hospitals solicited in their study of inpatient assaults refused to participate, presumably due to the risk of being a "high assault" hospital. Allowing assault levels to go unmeasured and unreported continues the denial of this issue and impedes the allocation of resources necessary to address the problem of patient assaults and clinician safety.

Architectural and Technical Strategies

Once there is an administrative and political awareness of the issue of patient violence and clinician safety, it is possible to proceed with concrete strategies to enhance clinician safety.

On inpatient wards, the geography of the units should be constructed to minimize blind corners. Traffic patterns to the dayroom or eating area should be assessed and appropriate space accorded so that patients are not required to be "herded together" at times of group activity such as meals. The nursing station should be constructed so as to provide a maximal view of the unit and ready access to, particularly, those parts of the unit where the highest patient density will be found.

The construction material for such units should minimize danger to staff. Shatterproof Plexiglas should be employed in windows of the nursing station (if the station is partially enclosed) and in the windows of the seclusion rooms. Despite some state regulations to the contrary, seclusion room doors should open outward to prevent their being barricaded shut or being used to trap a staff person within the seclusion room. Convex mirrors can be installed within seclusion rooms so that no blind corners exist where a patient might hide from a staff member, forcing the staff person to open the seclusion room and enter without knowing the precise location of the patient.

Dangerous furniture should be minimized on units where potentially violent patients are likely to be hospitalized. For example, heavy ashtrays or easily thrown chairs should be replaced. Commercial sand-filled chairs (Nemschoff Chairs, Inc., Sheboygan, Wisconsin) or heavy wooden chairs (Interroyal Corp., Plainfield, Connecticut) can be utilized that cannot be thrown. Lighting fixtures should be recessed or at least out of reach. They should be designed so that, if broken, they do not provide ready access to shards of glass that can be used as weapons. On highly assaultive units, pool balls can be replaced with Nerf balls for safety. On less restrictive units or activities therapy sites, access to knives or hammers and other potential weapons must be carefully monitored.

Additional technology can be superimposed onto wards for added safety. If blind spots do exist on a unit, or nursing staff is limited and cannot be in the dayroom all of the time, then either auditory or visual monitoring could be installed. For example, a closed-circuit television could be installed to monitor the dayroom on a ward where the room was at a significant distance from the nursing station. There is, nevertheless, a caveat for such monitoring, which is that staff must be designated as the *monitors* for such a system. A monitoring system in operation without someone systematically, frequently, and regularly monitoring the system provides a false sense of security that may, in fact, be more dangerous than having no monitoring system in operation at all.

Units with a high frequency of assault can also have built onto the wards individual alarm systems that can be carried by the ward staff. These alarms are connected to sensors distributed throughout the ward, wired through a wiring system that parallels the telephone wiring system. When activated by a staff member, these alarms can signal the ward's nursing station but can also be linked to a hospital-wide alarm network to provide outside assistance (described later). Several examples of alarm systems include the ET 2 linear transmitter (UNENCO, San Leandro, California), the Alarm Pen (Sentry Products, Santa Clara,

California), and other alarm systems (Lifeline Systems, Inc., Watertown, Massachusetts). Some can be activated by movement from a vertical to a horizontal position (when a staff member falls or is knocked to the ground) and do not need to be activated by the staff member.

In the emergency room, the setting for the assessment and management of potentially violent patients is also critical. Often "disturbing" patients either are seen in the middle of the very busy emergency room (to enhance visibility) or are placed far away from the medical emergencies (out of sight, out of mind?). Both of these options are less than ideal. With the first option, the setting is intense and overstimulating. The physical environment for the agitated patient should be an environment that assists in the de-escalation (i.e., quieting) of the patient, not in stimulating him or her further. In the latter case, placing an evaluation room away from central traffic patterns and staffing raises the risk of isolating staff and reducing the likelihood that they could obtain additional assistance if needed swiftly and certainly.

Evaluation rooms need to be large enough so that physical restraint, if necessary, can be implemented. Space for five staff members must be available as well as floor or gurney space to place an individual in a prone or supine position during restraint. Training should be given to clinicians to avoid their entering such rooms without informing other staff or, worse yet, locking themselves in such a room with a patient. The following example highlights the risks involved in such an action:

> A consulting neurologist was asked to see a mentally retarded young man on a locked psychiatric unit at a county hospital. The neurologist had the young man enter a small, confined examining room that had a self-locking door (presumably to keep patients from entering the room unattended). The neurologist proceeded with his examination and turned out the lights in this unfamiliar room to examine the patient's fundi. The patient, fearful of this action, physically attacked the neurologist. They rolled about the tiny room in the dark. Ward staff, hearing the commotion, were delayed in entering the room because it was locked. Eventually they entered, turned on the lights, and quieted the patient. The neurologist was significantly beaten but fortunately did not sustain any fractures or sutureable lacerations.

Rooms for psychiatric evaluation should also be devoid of "medical weapons." Often, to conserve emergency care space, a special procedures room doubles for the psychiatric assessment room. These areas frequently have glassware for suction and sharp and even heavy instruments for orthopedic procedures. Handled by a disturbed patient, such medical equipment can become a lethal weapon.

> A psychiatrist was asked to see a paranoid patient at the local hospital for an evaluation. The available room was the orthopedic room. During the assessment, the patient emotionally escalated and began to threaten the psychiatrist, asking him to leave. The psychiatrist continued to attempt to quiet the patient and did not leave. The patient grabbed a readily available orthopedic bar, attacked the psychiatrist, and clubbed him to death.

Safer environments in both situations could have led to substantially different outcomes.

Visual and auditory monitoring within the emergency room is also feasible but often overlooked in design. Although privacy in the patient interview is necessary, it is possible to design a sound-attenuated room that still has windows that allow for continuous monitoring of the staff and patient inside but ensure auditory privacy. During a more threatening interview, such rooms could utilize additional auditory monitoring through a speaker system that would connect to the nursing station. All rooms could be equipped either with special "code" buttons or a single-button telephone alarm system that would activate a behavioral emergency response (described later). Ideally, such behavioral assessment rooms would also have more than one door so that a clinician could exit even if the patient was obstructing one exit from the room.

Some high-volume emergency rooms, or emergency rooms in particularly violent areas, have adopted the use of metal detectors. As alluded to by Hartwig (Chapter 1, this volume) discussing ethics, the assault on personal dignity and the implied dangerousness of the emergency room environment have dissuaded some institutions from using these instruments. For sites that frequently have armed patients, the response toward safety may preempt the issues of respect and ambience.

The Veterans Administration, since the psychiatry directorship of Dr. Jack Ewalt, encouraged its hospitals to maintain a "flag" system for repetitively or seriously assaultive patients (assaultive either to themselves or others). The red or orange dot that appeared on the patient's record could be easily overlooked and often arrived too late—after violence had already occurred in the waiting area. On computerization of the registration system within the Veterans Administration, another option surfaced. In this case, "tickler" messages could be inserted in the computer record of veterans that would appear when they registered at the clinic using their Veterans Administration record number. Such ticklers could indicate, for example, that the patient was frequently, repetitively, or seriously assaultive. This would allow the staff to take immediate precautionary steps. Such interventions might be to request hospital security to come to the urgent care area until the patient had been evaluated. It might only encourage a speedy evaluation of the veteran so that he was not required to wait and potentially escalate, behaviorally, in the emergency room area. As reported by Drummond and colleagues (1989), such a computer system in the Portland Veterans Administration Hospital significantly reduced violent behavior in a repetitively violent patient group.

Finally, clinicians' individual offices need to be safe for the clinician as well. Once more, the caveat of having safe furniture and decorations obtains here as well. Ashtrays and statuary that can become weapons may be attractive, but they are also dangerous. As with the emergency room, double entrance and exit rooms offer additional safety and reduce the risk of entrapment. Although home offices offer much in the way of convenience and, perhaps, a tax advantage, they should be offices for only the safest of patients, since they are at a location often without other professional support and also put family at risk of exposure to a dangerous patient.

Institutional outpatient sites should be constructed so that there is both a physical and personal buffer for the clinician. Patients coming to see the clinician should first report in to a receptionist. This individual should be trained in assessing the emotional state of the patient and rehearsed in what action to take if the patient appears dangerous. Violent patients in such a situation, by history, generally appear intent on violence to the *clinician* and leave the receptionist alone. Such buffering can be lifesaving (if heeded). Annis and Baker (1986) described a physician's death under just these conditions:

> A chronic patient returned to a state hospital to see his previous therapist. He appeared in the antrum to the psychiatrist's office with a shotgun and requested from the secretary that he be allowed to see the

> psychiatrist. The secretary rang the psychiatrist and informed him that Mr. X. was waiting outside his office to see him *and* that Mr. X. was armed with a shotgun. Despite this buffering and warning, the psychiatrist opened the door and reached out to greet the patient, who immediately opened fire, killing the psychiatrist.

The buffer area and receptionist configuration can also be used for obtaining assistance. Prior codes can be worked out between a clinician and the secretary so that key remarks, such as "Please bring me Mr. Smith's orange chart" or "Would you tell me the time of my Code Orange meeting," can instruct a receptionist to call for the police or to initiate a behavioral emergency code.

Clinics where assaultive patients are seen should develop an alerting system. This can be a single-button alert that works through the telephone line or a separate "panic button" that can be attached in an inconspicuous location within reach of the therapist. Staff should practice their responses to the deployment of such alerts so that they are prepared if intervention is needed. Although administrators often balk at the cost of implementing such systems, they frequently will relent when the cost of a wrongful death lawsuit is presented in comparison.

Behavioral Intervention Plans

All clinician groups from the small group practice to the large state psychiatric hospital can (and probably should) maintain an active behavioral intervention plan. For a two- or three-clinician office, this may simply be a strategy to notify the other partner(s) of a need for assistance and to have the receptionist telephone the police.

For other mental health centers, general hospitals, or psychiatric hospitals, the system should be a more elaborate. Two examples can illustrate this point. The Veterans Administration hospital in Madison, Wisconsin, is a 200-bed general medical hospital with approximately 20 psychiatric beds. It has an urgent care area and will receive psychiatrically disturbed patients, intoxicated patients, but also patients agitated from organic disorders (e.g., from anesthesia, fever, or medication). This hospital has a behavioral emergency code system (Code Orange) that can be triggered by panic buttons in the urgent care area, the inpatient psychiatric unit, or the outpatient mental hygiene clinic. Code Orange can also be phoned to the page operator. Initiation of this system produces a response of five trained *site-designated* personnel to the point of origin of the code: 1) the medical officer of the day, 2) the nursing supervisor (at night) or psychiatry resident (during the day), 3) a psychiatric nurse from the inpatient psychiatry unit (who brings a "crash box" with restraints and intramuscular medications), 4) the administrative assistant from the urgent care area, and 5) a hospital police officer. This is a sufficient number to effect a five-person ambulatory restraint take down if necessary. Often this number of staff is simply required to provide an adequate "show of force" to encourage adherence to limits by the patient without escalation to violence. Staff in each of these positions are trained in verbal and physical intervention skills. They function in accordance with a hospital policy regarding the Code Orange, and all codes are reviewed in a quality assurance system developed by the psychiatry nurse specialist of the hospital. Such a system is geared for infrequent codes, perhaps one or two per month.

For busier programs, a more elaborate system is required. For example, at the 670-bed Dorothea Dix Hospital in Raleigh, North Carolina, a system labeled PIC (Preventive Intervention Course) has been developed. All psychiatric personnel are required to take and pass a formal training course in PIC, which includes lessons and practice in talking down and taking down violent patients. Training in verbal techniques is for 7 hours. Training in physical techniques also is for 7 hours. These training modules are repeated annually for the staff.

Once trained, staff is prepared to respond to PIC Minor and PIC Major codes throughout the hospital. These are triggered by telephone alerts to the hospital page operator or, on high-frequency assault units (the forensic unit and the management unit), by an automatic alarm system. When a PIC Minor is called, staff from adjacent wards are required to respond. When a PIC Major is called, it signals that a major assault is already in progress. Although adjacent units may respond, this alert requires the response of a team from the forensic unit, the members of which are even more highly trained in physical restraint. All PIC interventions are reviewed through a quality assurance mechanism to assess the appropriateness and effectiveness of the intervention.

Personal Training

All of the above interventions have been of a systems nature. Clinician safety can also be enhanced by individual training. As indicated by

Fink (Chapter 4, this volume), training can be implemented at the resident level and should be enhanced beyond what is currently being taught. Training can also be implemented through continuing medical education programs and grand rounds, where clinician safety is made a significant and timely issue. Continuing medical education courses can be taken at national meetings. For many years, such courses on managing the violent patient have been given at the American Psychiatric Association, and for the past several years the association's Task Force on Clinician Safety has held an annual workshop on managing patient interactions that could jeopardize clinician safety. Commercial courses in Akido are often given in large cities and can be taken to increase physical responsiveness. For institutions, consultant programs such as the program of the National Crisis Prevention Institute (Milwaukee, Wisconsin) can be contracted with to provide physical training for hospital staff.

Such programs offer a body of knowledge that can become a useful resource for the clinician when faced with a potentially dangerous clinical situation. Although a full exposition of this material exceeds the space available in this chapter, elements of it can be reviewed.

First, clinicians must maintain a high suspicion for violent behavior in their patient population. Although certain predictors of violence exist—such as a history of violence, intoxication, active threats, access to weapons, social isolation, psychotic mentation, suicidal ideation, or pathological interaction with a potential victim (unpublished VA Guidelines, 1976)—these paradoxically pose more of a risk for the clinician if one's guard is dropped for patients who do not meet these criteria. In Tardiff's (1983) review of assaultive behavior in psychiatric inpatients, one conclusion that can be drawn is that delusionally and otherwise psychotic individuals pose the greatest risk of assault. However, the study also demonstrated that patients in essentially any diagnostic group can manifest assaultive behavior. Similarly, the expectation is that involuntarily hospitalized patients are those to be watched for assaultive behavior, yet 51% of all clinician assaults in the study by Hatti and colleagues (1982) occurred with outpatients. In a subsequent survey by Dubin and colleagues (1988), 36% of outpatient assaults occurred with patients who had been in therapy with the clinician for longer than 1 year.

A tragic clinical vignette can serve to illustrate this selective denial.

A second-year psychiatry resident at a training program based at a university hospital and at the affiliated Veterans Administration Hospital had been a part of a resident's lobby to increase safety at the Veterans Administration. At this hospital, a behavioral emergency program had been put into effect. Buzzers had been placed in the emergency care's interview room and in the outpatient clinic. Hospital police had been trained to respond to the request of psychiatry residents who felt uncomfortable interviewing threatening Vietnam veterans. Yet, it was at the university clinic where this resident saw a young schizophrenic male off medication before clinic hours, alone in her office. It was at the university where this young man, once inside the office, pulled a .22 handgun and shot and killed the resident and himself. There was significant speculation during the psychological autopsy that followed that this resident would not have behaved in this manner had the patient appeared at the Veterans Administration Hospital, where the expectation of violence was actually higher.

A lowered index of suspicion can "join hands" with the clinician's sense of denial. Even after serious threats or assaults, clinicians may adopt a "conspiracy of silence," a cloak of denial. In their study of outpatient violence, Dubin and colleagues (1988) noted that 21% of the time, clinicians who continued to treat the assaultive patient failed to discuss with their patient the assault that occurred in their office. A similar error can be made by the clinician failing to share threats, the development of a psychotic transference, or other signals of an unsafe clinical situation with professional peers or consultants to broaden the awareness of the situation and enlist further clinical expertise. I have already illustrated the coupling of grandiosity with denial in the case reported by Annis and Baker (1986) cited earlier. The interpersonal skills of psychiatric clinicians tragically and repetitively are demonstrated to be inadequate to the unpredictability, psychoses, and anger of a subpopulation of our patients. Hence, dispelling our denial and our grandiosity will go a long way in enhancing our personal safety, especially when coupled to an alert awareness that almost any patient of ours has the potential for violence.

Beyond this psychological set, and a sensitivity to the signs of behavior escalating toward violence (Tardiff 1989), there are some basic tenets of managing aggressive patients as well as defensive techniques of verbal, physical, and even chemical intervention that can be helpful in reducing the probability of clinician assault (Eichelman 1991).

Basic tenets in the management of the violent patient must begin with training for the clinician. This then leads to control of the clinical situation, followed by diagnosis and assessment, and finally to treatment and management. If this progression is taken out of order, the risk of violent and assaultive behavior increases. Linked to this linear way of proceeding to manage the violent patient are three overarching management principles: 1) to strive to decrease tension in the potentially violent situation, 2) to attempt to *prevent* the violent episode, and 3) to function as a clinical team.

Psychological autopsies or even training role playing may serve to illustrate how unwittingly therapists may increase tension in the therapeutic interaction with the use of threatening body language, loud speech, or the setting of unnecessary limits. Similar review of ward violence may illustrate how ward personnel at times wait until the patient is out of control and actually assaultive before intervening. An escalating patient is a behavioral emergency just as severe chest pain is a cardiac emergency. Intervention (e.g., the use of a time-out or a prn medication) *before* the assault is the appropriate intervention. Lastly, violence reduction and assault reduction are team efforts. The control of a threatening patient will, in all likelihood, require the participation of several individuals to control the situation. Limit setting by one individual who may not be able to enforce the limit (e.g., the 5-foot female nurse who tells the 250-pound combat-trained veteran that he cannot leave the ward) becomes a high-probability situation for assault. In contrast, the use of a show-of-force team (see later) can reduce the ambiguity of limit enforcement and reduce the risk of violence.

The violent or threatening patient may require the use of consultants or a whole clinic's or group's response to protect the targeted clinician. In certain situations, delusional and threatening patients should be transferred to other therapists or even a therapy team to diffuse a pathological transference. Team approaches may bridge professional lines. Under certain circumstances of threat, other agencies should clearly be involved. Serious threats may require notification of law enforcement agencies for protection. Even legal remedies such as restraining orders or refusal to treat at a particular institution or program may be the appropriate response to decrease the risk of assaultive behavior directed at a targeted clinician.

Verbal and Interpersonal Strategies

Particularly in the "control" phase of patient management, or in the situation where a patient's aggression is escalating, several behavioral strategies can be used to reduce the risk of clinician assault.

First, clearly identify yourself as a clinician. Particularly in the emergency room with delirious or intoxicated patients, the clinician may be mistaken for someone outside of the helping role. In this regard, it may be useful to utilize a "white coat style" while assessing such disordered patients. Clear identification with the "medical role" may for some patients call forth some inhibition of assaultive behavior. In addition to visual cues, in such situations, the clinician needs to repeat over and over again his or her intentions and purpose in the verbal interaction because such information simply may not be attended to by a patient who is emotionally aroused.

Second, keep the proper physical distance. Approaching too rapidly and too closely to a disturbed patient may precipitate an assault. Behavioral studies (Kinzel 1970) indicate that individuals with an assaultive history have a larger "body buffer zone" than nonassaultive individuals. Moreover, this zone is larger behind than in front of the individual. A general guidance would be to be "two quick steps" from the patient—close enough to move to physical restraint, if necessary, but distant enough to avoid a physical attack. When approaching the patient, approach from in front or the front and side, not from behind.

Third, while keeping the proper physical distance, attempt to approximate the body language of the patient in ways that "meet" the patient's affect and energy but strive to de-escalate the situation. Thus, a standing patient should be met standing, but if the patient is pacing and speaking loudly, the clinician should model a slower walk and a slightly lower voice, which can lead the patient to a decreased state of tension. However, the disparity between patient and clinician cannot be too great. The shouting patient and the whispering therapist will, in all probability, lead to further escalation because the patient will not feel that the clinician has emotionally "met" him or her as regards affect. The sitting patient should be interviewed by a seated clinician whose body language models openness and candor—with a posture that is open and not marked by folded arms or tightly crossed legs.

Fourth, use "active" listening. Emotionally distraught patients require a response from a clinician that transcends the analyst's "Uh, huh, tell me more." Active eye contact and body language that signal attentiveness and connectedness to the patient will reduce the probability that the patient will need to "explode" or assault to get his or her point across.

Fifth, make use of the active-listening technique of paraphrasing: say back to the patient in brief encapsulated form the content of his or her statements (e.g., "Yes, I understand that you are so angry you feel like you could shoot your brother. I hear you can do it, that you have a loaded gun in the car.") However, because most affectively aroused patients will need to ventilate their history, the clinician should not overly intrude into the interview. Perhaps a reasonable rule of thumb would be for the clinician to be speaking no more than 10 seconds out of every minute of the interview. More than this raises the risk that the patient will escalate further to be heard—perhaps leading to assault.

Finally, it is necessary to be impeccably precise and honest when responding to the patient. Precision can define the situation so that the individual may not need to "lose control" to get an appropriate clinical response. For example, often the patient in the emergency room is told that he or she must wait to be seen until the psychiatrist finishes up on the ward. This is not a precise statement and in its ambiguity (as with the 5-foot nurse) becomes a precipitant for violence. The patient knows—consciously or unconsciously—that by becoming violent he or she will get a more rapid response from the hospital staff. This may lead to a violent outburst. An alternative response would be for the clinician to inform the patient that he or she will be down to see the patient in 20 minutes, after finishing work with another patient on the ward. If there is any problem in making that deadline, the clinician will call and speak directly to the patient. Assuming the clinician respects the 20-minute contract, the patient does not need to escalate his or her aggressive behavior to be seen.

Similarly, dishonesty may set the clinician up for either retribution or at the very least a shaky subsequent therapeutic relationship. The clinician who promises "no medication" or "discharge in 72 hours" may be making promises that cannot be kept. Respect for the patient requires integrity on the part of the clinician even if this moves the relationship into issues of resistance leading to seclusion and restraint.

Physical Strategies

Physical strategies include the environment, alarms, a show of force, behavioral response teams, seclusion, and restraint. As a physical strategy, the environment has already been discussed. A safe environment should be one free from potential weapons. It should be an area that reduces rather than enhances stimulation. It should be large enough to allow for the admission of a behavioral emergency team should one be necessary and for the immobilization of the patient if indicated. It should have easy entrance and egress.

Alarms as a physical strategy have also been discussed. Visual and auditory monitoring can serve an alarm function; so, too, can metal detectors, computer-programmed "ticklers," and personal or strategically located panic buttons.

However, alarms are only as effective as the behavioral response that follows. As discussed earlier, trained behavioral emergency teams within the hospital or clinic setting and well-rehearsed plans for the small group practice can, when effectively implemented, greatly reduce the probability of clinician injury. Such behavioral teams allow for the enforcement of limit setting through a show of force or, if necessary, can execute a humane and rapid physical restraint.

The guidelines and techniques for seclusion and physical restraint are beyond the scope of this chapter. They have been reviewed elsewhere (American Psychiatric Association 1985). Nevertheless, restraint, in particular, should be mentioned as a technique to reduce clinician injury. Just as sailing ahead full sail is hazardous in the middle of a storm, so, too, is attempting to diagnose and treat the patient who is out of control. Not only may medical conditions be missed, but the assessor may also become a victim in the attempt to intervene. The sequence is control, diagnose, and treat. Control must come first.

Pharmacological Strategies

As the psychopharmacology for the treatment of aggressive patients has evolved, the sophisticated use of medication has become yet another strategy that can be used to manage the aggressive patient, and, in turn, reduce the risk of clinician assault. Medication can be utilized both as chemical restraint and as a long-term treatment agent. Classes of drugs utilized in the chemical-restraint situation for the out-of-control patient include barbiturates, benzodiazepines, and high-potency antipsychotic agents. At present, there are few data to suggest one class of agent over another. However, particularly for psychotic patients, a combination of an antipsychotic agent and a benzodiazepine has been reported as quite beneficial in controlling the acute agitation of newly admitted psychiatric patients (Salzman et al. 1986).

In the longer term treatment of assaultive patients with psychopharmacologic agents, it is worthwhile to restate some guidelines for such treatment. First, in the pharmacologic treatment of repetitively assaultive patients, some form of assessment or rating mechanism should be in place to determine the success or failure of a medication. This could be the use of a rating scale such as the Overt Aggression Scale (Yudofsky et al. 1986), designed for inpatient assessment. Second, such treatment should have a beginning and an end—a point when the efficacy of the agent is assessed. If the agent is ineffective, it is discontinued. Third, if violence occurs in a patient with a specific psychiatric disorder, medication should initially be targeted for that primary disorder. Last, if "innovative" medications are going to be used, agents such as carbamazepines, beta blockers, or serotonin-enhancing drugs, begin with the less dangerous drugs in a systematic trial and move to increasingly more dangerous drugs. A discussion of specific pharmacologic agents is beyond the scope of this chapter. Such reviews are available elsewhere (Eichelman 1986).

Summary

In this chapter, I have attempted to lead the reader along many paths to already known political, administrative, architectural, psychological, behavioral, and chemical interventions that can be learned by the clinician and implemented in his or her practice. An increased awareness of clinician safety coupled with the systematic application of such strategies will reduce clinician violence.

References

American Psychiatric Association: Seclusion and Restraint: The Psychiatric Uses (Task Force Report No 22). Washington, DC, American Psychiatric Association, 1985

Annis LV, Baker CA: A psychiatrist murder in a mental hospital. Hosp Community Psychiatry 37:505–506, 1986

Drummond DJ, Sparr LF, Gordon GH: Hospital violence reduction among high-risk patients. JAMA 261:2531–2534, 1989

Dubin WR, Wilson SJ, Mercer C: Assaults against psychiatrists in outpatient settings. J Clin Psychiatry 49:338–345, 1988

Eichelman B: Toward a rational pharmacotherapy for aggressive and violent behavior. Hosp Community Psychiatry 39:31–39, 1986

Eichelman B: Psychiatric mental health nursing with the violent patient, in Psychiatric Mental Health Nursing. Edited by Gary F, Kavanagh C. Philadelphia, PA, JB Lippincott, 1991, pp 900–920

Hatti S, Dubin WR, Weiss KJ: A study of circumstances surrounding patient assaults on psychiatrists. Hosp Community Psychiatry 33:660–661, 1982

Kinzel AF: Body-buffer zone in violent prisoners. Am J Psychiatry 127:99–104, 1970

Reid WH, Bollinger MF, Edwards JG: Assaults in hospitals. Bull Am Acad Psychiatry Law 13:1–4, 1985

Salzman C, Green AI, Rodriguez-Villa F, et al: Benzodiazepines combined with neuroleptics for management of severe disruptive behavior. Psychosomatics 27(suppl):17–21, 1986

Tardiff K: A survey of assault by chronic patients in a state hospital system, in Assaults Within Psychiatric Facilities. Edited by Lion JR, Reid WH. New York, Grune & Stratton, 1983, pp 3–19

Tardiff K: Assessment and Management of Violent Patients. Washington, DC, American Psychiatric Press, 1989

Yudofsky SC, Silver JM, Jackson W, et al: The overt aggression scale for the objective rating of verbal and physical aggression. Am J Psychiatry 143:35–39, 1986

Chapter 11

Prosecution as a Response to Violence by Psychiatric Patients

Kenneth L. Appelbaum, M.D., and Paul S. Appelbaum, M.D.

Little is known about the historical incidence of assaults against mental health professionals (Ekblom 1970). Aggressive behavior by patients toward their treatment providers probably has always occurred, but attempts to assess the frequency of assaults have encountered methodological problems. Studies relying on incident reports from psychiatric hospitals (Evenson et al. 1974; Kalogerakis 1971) have been criticized by other investigators (Lion et al. 1981; Tardiff and Sweillam 1982) who have found higher rates of assaults after more exhaustive reviews of hospital records. One survey of therapists found that 24% had been attacked during 1 year by one or more patients (Whitman et al. 1976). In another survey, 42% of psychiatrists reported having been assaulted by a patient at some time in their careers (Madden et al. 1976). In both surveys, attacks were not limited to professionals with hospital-based practices but included private practitioners and community psychiatrists as well.

Although assaults against therapists are not a new phenomenon, it is likely that their frequency, at least in inpatient settings, is increasing. The population of hospitalized psychiatric patients includes a growing proportion of persons who display chronic character pathology and violent behavior (Johansen 1983). At least three factors may partly account for this trend. First, some categories of deviant behavior have been reclassified as indicators of mental illness suitable for psychiatric hospitalization and treatment (Melick et al. 1979; Reich 1981). As a result, some studies suggest, a higher percentage of patients with prior criminal histories are being admitted to psychiatric hospitals (Steadman et al. 1978). Second, the potential malpractice liability of psychiatrists for an outpatient's violent acts has expanded with the 1976 *Tarasoff* decision by the California Supreme Court. Psychiatrists consequently may feel constrained to hospitalize and detain persons judged to be dangerous to others, regardless of their appropriateness for inpatient treatment (P. S. Appelbaum 1984, 1988). There are some preliminary data to suggest that this may, in fact, be occurring (Lidz et al. 1989; Turkington 1986). Third, the shift from "need for treatment" to a "dangerousness" criterion for civil commitment has further skewed the inpatient population toward a more violent composition. Nondangerous mentally ill persons, who do not meet civil commitment criteria, may be denied voluntary admission, especially to public sector facilities, where limited resources tend to be reserved for committable patients. Although only a minority of involuntary patients are admitted solely because of danger to others (Hoge et al. 1989; Monahan et al. 1982), this group represents a higher proportion of patients than was previously the case and appears to contribute disproportionately to the violence occurring on inpatient units (McNiel and Binder 1987).

The growing awareness of the problem of assaults on psychiatric staff has led to intensified efforts to find appropriate means of preventing and responding to such assaults. Among the suggested responses to patients' violence is the use of criminal prosecution, which has been the subject of several writings. The first case involving prosecution was reported in 1978 (Schwarz and Greenfield 1978). Since then, another 15 cases of filing criminal charges against psychiatric patients for assaults on staff or other patients have appeared in four additional reports (Hoge and Gutheil 1987; Miller and Maier 1987; Norko et al. 1992; Phelan et al. 1985). Under what circumstances is filing criminal charges against a patient indicated or justified? What are the likely effects of prosecution? How should the decision to press charges be made? In an attempt to answer these questions, we examine the justifications for criminal sanctions, relevant issues of professional ethics, a clinical approach to making these decisions, and practical considerations if prosecution is pursued.

Justifications for Criminal Sanctions

Prosecution of patients for violent behavior must rely for its justification, in part, on the same rationales that underpin the imposition of criminal sanctions in general. Before considering the unique problems raised by resorting to prosecution in a therapeutic environment, therefore, it is necessary to review the purposes for, and justifications of, prosecution in the broader criminal context.

The goal of criminal prosecution is the imposition of sanctions against offenders who are judged guilty of a criminal act. These sanctions, in turn, serve the ultimate purpose of either intentional infliction of suffering on wrongdoers or prevention of crime. Although further delineation is possible, in the final analysis, all justifications for criminal punishment rely on one or the other of these goals. A more thorough examination of the purposes of prosecution, however, requires a discussion of four specific models. These are retribution, deterrence, incapacitation, and rehabilitation (Packer 1968).

Retribution

According to the theory of retribution, it is proper to mete out punishment to someone who has broken the law. This has nothing to do with attaining revenge, as that term is usually understood, in that the emotional satisfaction of the agent inflicting punishment or of society in general is irrelevant to the purpose of the retributive response. Rather, the criminal, who has violated the terms of the social contract, must, for the sake of fairness to the other parties to that contract, be made to suffer the agreed-on penalty for his or her transgression. It is frequently said, in this regard, that convicted criminals receive their "just deserts." In general, the retributive point of view looks backward. It concerns itself with the crime already committed and not with future possibilities. Prevention of crime is not a consideration.

There is, however, an additional argument sometimes made to bolster the retributive approach. That argument maintains that state-sponsored retribution is necessary to satisfy the animosity of the populace toward the offender. If criminals are not punished by the state in proportion to their crimes, then victims' desires for vengeance remain unfulfilled. Individuals might then seek their own form of justice to the ultimate detriment of the social order. This argument attempts to provide a practical, forward-looking justification for the retributive point of view. Strict retributionists, however, eschew such pretexts.

Deterrence

In contrast to theories predicated on the intentional infliction of suffering, most justifications for criminal sanctions rely on one or another model of prevention. Perhaps foremost among them is the doctrine of deterrence. Two distinct types of deterrence are usually recognized. The first type of deterrence, *general* deterrence, refers to the ability of law enforcement to foster law-abiding behavior by all citizens in the society. This is accomplished primarily in three ways. First, the threat of apprehension and punishment for a crime, if certain and severe enough, will outweigh the potential rewards. Public awareness of successful prosecution and sanctioning of offenders serves to highlight this perception. Second, moral inhibitions against unlawful behavior are strengthened by the educational effects of criminal punishment. By conveying society's disapproval of an act, prosecution has a socializing influence that promotes the internalization of societal norms. Third, both moral inhibitions and fear of punishment encourage the development of lawful habits of behavior. These learned behaviors are selected in an unconscious and automatic fashion. Some contend that habit, along with moral inhibition, represents the primary value of general deterrence. Unlike the threat of punishment, these factors constrain behavior even when detection of a criminal act is unlikely.

The second type of deterrence is *specific* deterrence. Rather than focusing on the general population, this concept emphasizes the effects of punishment on the person being punished. The actual consequences of prosecution are postulated to have an intimidating effect. Here, it is the individual's experience with received punishment that discourages further illegal activity. This involves the same mechanisms that affect the populace at large: fear of sanctions; moral conditioning, reinforced through the already felt stigma of criminal conviction; and formation of habits of lawful behavior.

There are limitations on the efficacy of deterrence, and the theory has been criticized on a number of grounds (Andenaes 1952). The prevalence of crime and the incidence of recidivism are pointed out as indicators of the failure of both general and specific deterrence. These conclusions overlook the fact that the actual effectiveness of deterrence cannot be measured. We simply do not know what the crime rate would be if the threat of punishment did not exist, any more than we know what would be the incidence of recidivism. It is also argued that deterrence exerts its influence mainly on those individuals who are already predisposed to be law abiding. Individuals who are not intimidated by the threat of punishment, either because of psychological impairments or already desperate social circumstances, will not refrain from criminal conduct. This is a valid contention, but it ignores the effects that deterrence itself may have on the formation of law-abiding attitudes among those who are yet malleable. An even more disturbing criticism focuses on the negative effects of incarceration. The often appalling conditions in prisons may breed resentment and antisocial feeling in inmates. Rather than intimidation, the net result can be deeper alienation and an increased likelihood of recidivism. Despite these limitations, deterrence remains a powerful justification for criminal sanctions.

Incapacitation

Although the efficacy of deterrence is difficult to determine, incarceration is a certain way of preventing, in the community, further criminal activity by known offenders for a fixed period. It effectively incapacitates the individual in his or her ability to behave in a criminal manner in the society at large. Penal detention reduces or eliminates the opportunities to commit many types of crime. The implicit assumption is that without confinement the criminal will commit other crimes if given the chance. In many instances, however, the validity of this prediction of recidivism is questionable. Some illegal acts are unlikely to be repeated. Other crimes may be habitual but relatively trivial (e.g., shoplifting). Effective incapacitation of these latter wrongdoers often requires societal resources markedly disproportionate to the offense. Ironically, incapacitation may be most useful for those offenders who are either the least remediable (e.g., sociopathic persons with multiple prior offenses) or the least blameworthy (e.g., patients who assault in response to fixed paranoid delusions). Nevertheless, incapacitation is a credible model of prevention in cases where other approaches, such as deterrence, fail and where reoccurrence of criminal activity is likely.

Rehabilitation

Reformation of the criminal offender as a goal of punishment is not a new idea. The doctrine's popularity has waxed and waned in parallel with theories that assume that the causes of human behavior can be identified and therapeutic measures can be employed to effect changes in behavior. According to this model, crime can be prevented if antisocial tendencies are modified through treatment of the offender. The focus, therefore, is on the needs of the criminal rather than the nature of the crime. The duration of punishment is determined by the time required to change the offender's behavior. In its purest form, rehabilitation involves indeterminate sentences and confinement until the criminal's dangerous propensities are eliminated.

Despite its periodic popularity, rehabilitation is not without its detractors (Allen 1964). Perhaps the most telling criticism is that the task exceeds the capabilities of the institutions of criminal law. In many instances, we do not understand the causes of antisocial behavior, and, when we do, the antecedents are often multifactorial with roots in the social structure, as well as in the individual. In short, punishment for the purpose of rehabilitation remains a largely unrealized ideal.

Criminal Sanctions in the Therapist-Patient Relationship: Ethical Issues

How do these justifications for criminal prosecution apply if the offender is a patient and the victim is the patient's therapist or another patient? Do additional factors need to be taken into account? For example, what effect should the fiduciary relationship between therapist and patient have on the decision to bring criminal charges? These questions cannot be answered without prior consideration of the psychiatrist's obligations to the offending patient, to other patients and society in general, and to staff.

Basic obligations of psychiatrists toward patients include beneficence, the affirmative duty to act in the patient's best interests; nonmaleficence, the duty to do no harm; and autonomy, the obligation to respect the patient's right to self-determination (Beauchamp and Childress 1983). These and other fundamental principles of biomedical ethics are only prima facie obligations. At times they may conflict with one another, as well as with competing responsibilities of the clinician to third parties. For example, in general, health professionals respect a patient's autonomy to refuse treatment even if the decision is not in the patient's best interest. In contrast, the principle of nonmaleficence, along with other considerations, would most likely preclude compliance with a competent patient's request for a harmful intervention. Similarly, the beneficent duty to protect third parties at risk from a patient's violent behavior will, at times, necessitate violating patient autonomy by disclosing confidential information without consent. Although one obligation may take precedence in specific instances of conflict, compelling reasons are required before any of these basic ethical duties are compromised. The following discussion illustrates some ways in which the decision to prosecute a patient impinges on each of these principles.

In considering a psychiatrist's ethical obligations, some commentators suggest the existence of an affirmative therapeutic responsibility to press charges against assaultive patients. They contend that prosecution is not only justifiable but also beneficial for patients (Schwarz and Greenfield 1978). Other clinicians recommend to community members who have been injured by patients' criminal acts that they press charges against disruptive patients if that action is determined to be in the patient's best clinical interests (Stein and Diamond 1985). Family members are sometimes urged to take the same course (Fine and Acker 1989). These points of view appear to blend the therapist's duty of beneficence with the rehabilitative ideal. The clinician unilaterally selects or recommends to third parties a course of treatment (i.e., prosecution), and the criminal justice system becomes the instrument of therapy. Other ethical obligations, however, are neglected by this approach. Lack of prior consultation with the patient constitutes a disregard of the principle of autonomy. The derivative right to informed consent requires the patient's involvement in the decision or recommendation to prosecute if that action is being justified on therapeutic grounds. In addition, the demands of nonmaleficence impose further problems on prosecution for treatment purposes. As previously noted, the capacity of our penal institutions to rehabilitate offenders has been grossly overrated. Incarceration in a correctional setting, if not prosecution itself, can be a brutalizing experience. The offender might come out embittered and changed for the worse rather than the better. Invoking the criminal process may harm patients far more than it helps them (Fine and Acker 1989).

Finally, it is misleading to think of "therapeutic prosecution" primarily as being for the benefit of the patient. In fact, those who recommend this approach acknowledge its value in setting limits and reducing the frequency of criminal behavior. Although prosecution might help patients by improving their social adjustment, their well-being is ultimately incidental to the underlying goal of benefiting society. Therapeutic prosecution, therefore, relies more on models of specific deterrence than it does on those of rehabilitation. Its principal goal is the prevention of further offenses. To pretend that the essential motivation is to help the offender involves specious logic. What is actually being imposed is punishment, based on a finding of criminal guilt. The good will of the staff cannot change this fact, nor can it alter the patient's accurate perception of the punitive aspects of prosecution. In sum, significant ethical problems arise if prosecution of patients is pursued for therapeutic purposes.

Nevertheless, there may be countervailing interests that outweigh ethical obligations to the patient in individual cases, legitimizing other grounds for the prosecution of patients. The existence of a psychiatrist's legal duty to protect third parties, for example, is well established. The *Tarasoff* case and its progeny are only one example of this duty (Beck 1985, 1990). The obligation may be even more compelling when the third party is also a patient in a psychiatric facility. In a 1988 court case, the Florida Department of Health and Rehabilitative Services was held to have a duty to warn a hospitalized patient that she would be exposed to another inpatient with a known history of assaultive behavior. The court also found that the department had an obligation to supervise adequately the assaultive patient and her victim (*McCall and McCall v. Department of Health and Rehabilitative Services* 1988).

The legal duty stems from the state's affirmative duty to protect confined persons from harm. The ethical basis for this legal duty is readily apparent. During hospitalization, patients have either voluntarily surrendered, or had taken from them against their will, the ability to protect themselves from assault by regulating their living situation and associations. They do this in exchange for an implicit—and sometimes explicit—promise that they will be helped by hospitalization and protected from harm. Thus, the duty of nonmaleficence applies unambiguously in this context to patients who may be injured by other patients' violence.

This duty can be met in a number of ways, such as those suggested elsewhere in this volume, for the reduction of the risk of violence. Unfortunately, however, psychiatry is ill equipped to deal with assaultive behavior that is not associated with an underlying treatment-responsive mental illness. There often are insufficient resources to supervise the growing number of hospitalized patients with histories of violence. Prosecution may, at times, represent the only potentially effective means of protecting other patients and staff and may, in those circumstances, be justifiable.

Another obligation to society that psychiatrists may have in this area has been suggested by some authors. They contend that "the public has a right to know about serious assaults, . . . the failure to file a police report deprives the public of that information . . . [and] professionals may have a duty to initiate charges in cases where a serious assault has occurred" (Phelan et al. 1985, p. 582). This proclaimed duty—apparently independent of any retributive goal—has been denounced as "dangerous nonsense" (Gutheil 1985). A course of action that violates confidentiality and causes undeniable harm to the patient certainly requires more compelling justification than a questionable right of the public to know. Many, if not most, serious assaults never become part of the public record. Some remain unreported, and the others are often diverted from prosecution at one of the many discretionary points in the criminal process. The police may elect not to make an arrest, the district attorney's office may choose not to institute charges, or the court may dispose of the case prior to an adjudication. In the absence of a comprehensive system for tracking all assaultive incidents and a vital social need for that information, there is no reason that similar discretion should not be exercised when deciding whether to report assaults that occur in psychiatric settings. In fact, the clinician's ethical obligations to the patient argue for even greater reluctance to report assaults when the only motivation to do so is the public's presumed right to know. Breaching confidentiality for this reason compromises, with insufficient justification, the psychiatrist's role as the patient's agent.[1]

---

[1]There is, however, a potential legal duty that confounds this issue. In a few states, statutes and case law exist that appear to require citizens to report felonies that come to their attention. Some statutes specifically refer to mental health personnel. Massachusetts law, for example, requires the superintendent of any state hospital or the director of any mental health facility of the department (of mental health) to report felonies "committed by or upon any person on the premises of the particular facility or by or upon any person in the care of the particular facility but not on the premises thereof" (Massachusetts General Laws 1987, Chapter 19, Section 10). In some states, failure to report can itself be the basis of misprision of a felony. Nevertheless, therapists are unlikely to be found criminally liable under this doctrine. In practice, misprision of a felony almost always requires that active assistance be provided to the felon. The passive failure to report, on its own, is unlikely to result in criminal charges (P. S. Appelbaum and Meisel 1986).

Might there be situations in which the psychiatrist owes allegiance only to society and incurs none of the traditional therapist-patient obligations? As mental health professionals, clinicians are called on to conduct evaluations that assist institutions of law. Mental health professionals may be asked to assess questions of competence to stand trial, criminal responsibility, or other legal issues. This forensic role differs from usual medical practice of acting in the patient's interest. Instead, expertise is offered to aid in the resolution of these legal questions. Clinicians function as agents of the state, and in these instances there is, in fact, no "patient" (Rappeport 1981). Most forensic psychiatrists would agree, however, that this does not allow the therapist to be totally devoid of responsibility to the persons evaluated. At a minimum, there is an obligation to inform the person being evaluated about the clinician's role and the limits, or absence, of confidentiality. In addition, many practitioners would refrain from nonessential disclosures that are likely to cause harm (P. S. Appelbaum 1985). Nevertheless, it might be argued that if the usual ethical obligations to the patient do not apply, then the decision whether to prosecute assaultive forensic "evaluees" may be unrestrained by the full demands of confidentiality, beneficence, and nonmaleficence. Although this argument may be valid for outpatient evaluees, hospitalized forensic evaluees may be patients in the sense that they are dependent for their care and well-being, and often for the treatment of their disorder, on the professional staff of the facility. Thus, the ethical analysis would appear to be similar for inpatient evaluees and for nonforensic patients.

A final ethical consideration involves obligations to staff members. Some mental health workers believe that being assaulted is part of the job (Lanza 1983). Others contend that in exchange for the authority to seclude and restrain patients, "staff accept some risk of assault without pressing charges against the patient" (Gutheil 1985, p. 1320). Psychiatric patients may be assaultive as a manifestation of their mental illness, and it seems appropriate that these individuals be dealt with clinically, if possible. But all violent behavior by patients cannot be attributed to psychiatric disturbance. Nonpsychotic motivations may underlie antisocial conduct despite the presence of a major mental illness. Even if one accepts the argument that violence coincident with the treatment of a disorder must be tolerated, unrelated violence certainly falls outside that rationale. The status of being a patient should not be construed as a license to offend with impunity.

For example, a patient who robs his therapist at gunpoint cannot persuasively demand confidentiality for the incident because it occurred during the therapy hour. Therapists' ethical obligations to patients do not necessarily require passive acceptance of criminal victimization. In addition, supervisors may have an affirmative obligation and legal duty to protect staff members from such assaults. If other means of protection are unlikely to succeed, under those circumstances, prosecution may become ethically defensible.

Applying the Ethical Analysis

If one accepts that the initiation of criminal charges[2] against patients by staff or therapists is ethically permissible under certain circumstances, then a way is needed to balance competing interests when choosing a course of action. An approach that takes into account the goals of prosecution may aid in making these decisions. Each of the following justifications for criminal sanctions can then be examined as it relates to clinical circumstances.

Retribution

Among all of the expressed purposes of criminal punishment, retribution alone is not based on utilitarian models but on the desire to confer "just deserts" on an offender. Two conflicting beliefs come into play when retribution is discussed: 1) that clinicians should not respond punitively to patients' behavior, thereby violating the duty of nonmaleficence; and 2) that, even so, some behaviors by patients are sufficiently outrageous that punishment seems appropriate. An example of the latter might be an attempt by a nonpsychotic patient to rape a hospital staff member. Can a set of principles be identified that would assist in selecting cases in which the usual rule of nonmaleficence would be set aside?

The task is a difficult one. The most salient consideration would appear to be whether the assaultive patient can be held responsible for his or her behavior. The criminal justice system has evolved a set of

---

[2]The filing of a civil action against a patient is not discussed within the scope of the chapter.

rules governing this determination, usually at issue when a defendant pleads "not guilty by reason of insanity." Such rules ordinarily focus on the defendants' ability to know or appreciate the wrongfulness of their acts or to conform their behavior to the requirements of the law. These rules reflect the common intuition that persons who commit offenses because of their mental illnesses—usually of psychotic intensity—should not be punished as a result.

Commentators in the limited literature on prosecution of patients have reflected similar ideas (Hoge and Gutheil 1987; Miller and Maier 1987; Norko et al. 1992). Yet, the means by which responsibility should be determined in clinical settings are not at all clear. Basing the determination on a formal forensic evaluation of criminal responsibility utilizing the jurisdiction's legal standard for culpability misses the point that responsibility is a social, not a medical, judgment (Halleck 1984). Courts, not clinicians, determine criminal responsibility. To attempt to mimic the judicial process is unjustified. It may also lead to legal complications at a later point in the process. For example, an evaluation based on the jurisdiction's legal standard for criminal responsibility might be used as inculpatory evidence by the prosecutor despite the evaluation's actual purpose of aiding only in the clinician's decision of whether to press charges against the patient.

Clinical decision making might better be based on a straightforward consideration of the degree to which the patient's behavior was motivated by his or her mental disorder, particularly at a psychotic level. The closer the link between psychosis and behavior, the less justifiable prosecution appears to be.

Yet, this is clearly not the end of the matter. Most clinicians appear to share the belief that the more serious the assaultive behavior, the lower the threshold should be for invoking retributive justifications. Thus, even with a psychotic patient whose illness may have provoked his or her actions, one would be more prone to file charges for a rape or attempted murder than for a simple assault. Can we justify this position? Perhaps as the seriousness of the violence increases, society's interest in the accuracy and fairness of the process used to determine whether retribution is forthcoming becomes greater. At some point, the clinician's duty of nonmaleficence toward a patient whose behavior is illness-induced gives way to society's right to make the determination of culpability.

Could it be argued that this is always the case, that is, that clinicians should always file charges and allow the courts to determine the level of the patient's responsibility? Although the desire for black-and-white rules in this area is understandable, this position would seem to go too far toward undermining the obligation of nonmaleficence. Some balance must be achieved, and an approach that looks both to the seriousness of the offense and its relation to the patient's mental disorder appears to be a reasonable basis for striking that balance.

A final factor ought to be taken into account as well. Retribution as a justification for seeking prosecution of assaultive patients is further weakened if prosecution would substantially interfere with the patient's treatment needs. For example, a patient with a major mental illness might be at greater risk of decompensation under the stress of incarceration. In addition, psychiatric services within jails are often limited or nonexistent. When criminal proceedings are likely to exacerbate seriously a patient's condition, then duties of nonmaleficence dictate that greater caution be exercised before pressing charges. This applies even in the presence of behavior due to deliberate criminal intent.

Although retribution cannot be excluded as a reason for prosecuting patients, it appears to be justifiable only in a narrow range of circumstances. As the relationship between a psychotic disorder and the assaultive act diminishes, and as the severity of the violence increases, the justification for prosecution on retributive grounds grows. The disruption of patients' treatment and consequent harm as a result of prosecution may also need to be taken into account.

Deterrence

What about deterrence as a justification for pressing charges against assaultive patients? There are occasions in the clinical setting when one patient serves as an instigator or negative role model for others in the initiation of violence, and his or her prosecution would inhibit the spread of additional violence. The general deterrent effect may be an additional consideration in the decision of whether to pursue criminal punishment, but it is not a sufficient justification in its own right. In the absence of other reasons to prosecute, the patient is being used merely as a means to control the behavior of others. This transgresses the therapeutic relationship between patient and clinician. Moreover, patients who assault in response to their psychoses are unlikely to be influenced by the spectacle of another patient's prosecution. Although general deterrence may be a valid argument for criminal sanctions as a whole, and even there the same problems arise, its results are certainly too indirect and tenuous to abrogate the unique ethical obligations of the therapist to the patient.

Specific deterrence, on the other hand, oriented toward changing the behavior of assaultive patients themselves, might be a reasonable and effective means of protecting third parties under certain circumstances. This is especially true when clinical attempts to modify a patient's assaultive behavior have been exhausted. The likelihood of successful deterrence, however, has to be considered in view of the many shortcomings of this model of prevention. The shortcomings of specific deterrence limit its persuasiveness as a justification for prosecution.

Incapacitation

Initiating the criminal process for the purpose of diverting assaultive patients to the control of the criminal justice or correctional systems might be warranted when clinical means are unavailable to protect other patients or staff. The most obvious example is the patient who is uncontrollable in the mental health system and threatens the continuing safety of others. This incapacitation rationale presupposes two conditions. First, all reasonable interventions (e.g., medication, supervision, restraint) have been unsuccessful or are not practical given existing resources. Second, prosecution is likely to result in placement of the offender in a more secure correctional institution that is not accessible to civilly committed patients. Successful diversion to a penal setting prevents further assaults in the psychiatric institution.

Rehabilitation

As previously noted, the concept of therapeutic prosecution is suspect. Most people do not personally benefit from their experiences with the criminal justice system. Although rehabilitation has at least as much to do with benefiting others as it does with benefiting the offender, incarceration in the current correctional system seems to be a poor means of preventing recidivism after release (although whether it might be more effective for mentally ill offenders has, to our knowledge, never been explored). As such, rehabilitation as a justification for prosecution is subject to constraints very similar to those that apply to specific deterrence. Clinical interventions should be attempted first, and, even when these are exhausted, the deficiencies of prosecution in preventing recidivism warrant consideration.

Practical Issues

Ethical appropriateness is only one factor to be considered in deciding whether to initiate criminal charges against patients for assaults. There are many impediments to successful prosecution, and the decision to invoke the criminal process has potentially undesirable consequences. The legal system is often reluctant to process these cases (Hoge and Gutheil 1987; Miller and Maier 1987; Norko et al. 1992), and, even when it does, the ultimate disposition may be an outcome unsatisfactory to the staff who initiate the action (Hoge and Gutheil 1987). In addition to resistance by the criminal justice establishment, other practical problems include untoward effects on the offender, other patients, staff, the mental health facility, and the law itself.

Successful prosecution requires the cooperation of police, prosecutors, courts, and correctional officials. The process is undermined if any of these parties fail to cooperate. Police must first determine the likelihood that a crime has been committed and establish probable cause for arrest. They may decline to arrest because of the absence of sufficient evidence for prosecution or because of their awareness of the suspect's psychiatric status. The American Bar Association (1989) admonishes police not to arrest mentally disturbed persons for minor criminal conduct. At the same time, the American Bar Association recommends:

> When a police officer has arrested a person for a felony or other serious crime . . . such person should be processed in the same manner as any other criminal suspect notwithstanding the fact that the arresting officer has reasonable grounds for believing that the person's behavior meets statutory and departmental guideline requirements for emergency detention for mental evaluation. (p. 40)

The association explains that in felony cases "which manifest a serious threat to human life and safety, immediate and secure custody has to be the primary objective of the criminal justice system" (p. 42). Thus, although the police clearly can exercise discretion in deciding when to arrest, this is primarily true in cases of minor offenses. If criminal complaints are reserved for more serious incidents, there is a greater likelihood that police will cooperate with mental health staff.

When the police do choose to make an arrest, the district attorney, after weighing the evidence and the circumstances of the alleged crime, can still decline to pursue the charges. This might be due to a reluctance to prosecute a psychiatric patient, the belief that a hospitalized patient is "right where he belongs," the perception that a civilly committed patient will not be confined longer if convicted of a crime, or the contention that being assaulted is part of a mental health professional's job. Curiously, this latter attitude that psychiatric facilities, by virtue of their dangerous clientele, are essentially "free-fire zones" in which patients have license to assault with impunity appears not to be paralleled by similar attitudes regarding the correctional setting. We know of no evidence to suggest that criminal acts committed by prison inmates, especially if correctional officers are the victims, are not vigorously prosecuted.

Even those cases that receive a court hearing may have an ultimately unsatisfactory disposition. The judge can dismiss the charges and even admonish staff for initiating a criminal process against a patient for whom punishment cannot be "morally justified" (*State v. Cummins* 1979). If the case goes to trial, the patient can be found incompetent to stand trial or not guilty by reason of insanity and returned to the mental health system. In addition to outright acquittal, pleading to reduced charges is a possibility. Conviction itself often results in either a suspended sentence or release on probation. Finally, in the event of conviction and a sentence of penal incarceration, the patient may still return to the mental health system on a transfer from the correctional system for psychiatric treatment.

Such outcomes can be minimized in several ways. In individual cases, establishing a record of criminal offenses by prior prosecution, even if the initial prosecution is ultimately unsuccessful, can increase the willingness of the legal system to process the patient for future offenses. For example, where a former charge resulted in a suspended sentence or probation, a subsequent conviction is more likely to receive harsher penalties (e.g., United States Sentencing Commission 1992). Furthermore, liaison and general educational activities with criminal justice personnel can increase their sensitivity to these issues and foster their cooperation when an actual situation arises. Nonetheless, since all of the justifications for prosecution are dependent on the determined pursuit of conviction, the existence of severe practical impediments must be added to the balance before a decision to file charges is made.

A harmonious relationship between the mental health and legal systems, leading to active prosecution and conviction, still does not guarantee an outcome beneficial to all. The effects on the prosecuted patient, for example, can be either beneficial or adverse. Desired consequences include prevention of further offenses via incarceration (incapacitation) or behavior modification (specific deterrence or rehabilitation). Some also might see benefit in compelled treatment as a condition of probation or while charges are held in abeyance. Other potential consequences, however, are less desirable. Unsuccessful prosecution might inspire some patients to commit additional assaults without fear of consequences. Patients who are prosecuted might drop out of treatment (Hoge and Gutheil 1987), in part because of the damage done to the therapeutic alliance (Gutheil 1985). Finally, in addition to possible exacerbation of a patient's psychiatric condition, incarceration can have corrupting and embittering effects on the patient that foster further antisocial behavior. The length of the sentence and the kind of facility in which it is served can be very different from what was anticipated by those who initiated criminal prosecution in the first place (Fine and Acker 1989).

Prosecuting a patient also can have effects on fellow patients. One benefit might be a safer milieu through the removal or deterrence of the assaultive individual and deterrence of violence in general. In addition, other patients might be reassured by the knowledge that staff are prepared to deal with the problem of violence by whatever means are necessary. On the other hand, patients can perceive the pursuit of criminal charges as an indication of staff hostility and of their impotence to respond to the situation clinically. The likely effect that prosecution will have on patients' trust in staff members also warrants consideration.

Although "successful" prosecution might foster a safer workplace, "failure" of the criminal process might ultimately encourage the very behavior that prosecution was intended to prevent. In addition, clinician participation in the legal proceedings can be a traumatic experience. This is true not only when the criminal justice system resists prosecution, but also if the staff members involved are ambivalent, even when prosecution is vigorously undertaken. Conscious and unconscious countertransference reactions to violent patients can affect how staff members respond (Lion and Pasternak 1973). To the extent that their motivations are unclear or conflicted, members of the staff are at risk of feeling ill at ease. Furthermore, once the process of prosecution is invoked, the course and outcome can be different from that which staff intended. For example, a prosecution intended to effect specific deterrence by means of a short jail term might result in imposition of a much more severe penalty. Consultation with senior clinicians might aid staff members in clarifying their motivations and the potential outcomes of their behavior in initiating the legal process. These factors demonstrate the importance of deciding in advance, with all involved staff members participating, on the goals of prosecution. Without consensus on these goals and their legitimacy, to proceed with prosecution is to invite guilt and dissension among staff members and ultimately among patients as well.

Initiating criminal action against assaultive patients also has implications for the mental health facility that is involved. The potential for negative publicity exists, for example, when an institution places itself in an adversarial stance with patients by sanctioning prosecution. Although this might not preclude prosecution, it is a factor for administrative concern. Partly for this reason, institutional policies and guidelines that address the decision to prosecute need to be developed. Such policies would also allow staff to know in advance whether their actions will comport with institutional expectations.

Finally, prosecuting patients can negatively affect the criminal justice system itself. This can occur when clinicians initiate criminal complaints against patients either for minor offenses or for "therapeutic" reasons. In the former instance, courts can be overburdened with relatively trivial matters. In the latter case, the primary purpose of the legal system is overlooked. The aim of criminal sanctions is not to provide an additional treatment option for psychiatry. Diverting the resources of the legal system toward this end impairs its ability to fulfill its actual mission (Allen 1964).

Conclusion

Assaults by psychiatric patients are a growing concern, especially in inpatient settings. Potential responses by staff members range from clinical management to initiating legal action against the offending patient. The traditional rationales for the criminal sanction—retribution, deterrence, incapacitation, and rehabilitation—are necessary, but not sufficient, justifications for prosecution in this context. Unique ethical obligations of the therapist to the patient—and to other patients and staff members—impose additional constraints. The acceptability of prosecution can be assessed by examining these duties within the context of each of the purposes of the criminal sanction. Clinicians also need to address the practical effects of utilizing the criminal justice system. Reluctance of the criminal justice system to process these cases can be lessened through proactive educational and liaison activities with law enforcement personnel. Consultation with colleagues can help to clarify the likely effects of prosecution on the offender, other patients, and members of the staff. Finally, institutional policies need to be promulgated to guide clinicians and administrators in making these difficult decisions (K. A. Appelbaum and Appelbaum 1991).

References

Allen FA: The Borderland of Criminal Justice. Chicago, IL, The University of Chicago Press, 1964

American Bar Association: Criminal Justice Mental Health Standards. Washington, DC, American Bar Association, 1989

Andenaes J: General prevention—illusion or reality? Journal of Criminal Law, Criminology, and Police Science 43:176–198, 1952

Appelbaum KA, Appelbaum PS: A model hospital policy on prosecuting patients for presumptively criminal acts. Hosp Community Psychiatry 42:1233–1237, 1991

Appelbaum PS: Hospitalization of the dangerous patient: legal pressures and clinical responses. Bull Am Acad Psychiatry Law 12:323–329, 1984

Appelbaum PS: Confidentiality in the forensic evaluation. Int J Law Psychiatry 7:67–82, 1985

Appelbaum PS: The new preventive detention: psychiatry's problematic responsibility for the control of violence. Am J Psychiatry 145:779–785, 1988

Appelbaum PS, Meisel A: Therapists' obligations to report their patients' criminal acts. Bull Am Acad Psychiatry Law 14:221–230, 1986

Beauchamp TL, Childress JF: Principles of Biomedical Ethics, 2nd Edition. New York, Oxford University Press, 1983

Beck J (ed): The Potentially Violent Patient and the Tarasoff Decision in Psychiatric Practice. Washington, DC, American Psychiatric Press, 1985

Beck J (ed): Confidentiality Versus the Duty to Protect: Foreseeable Harm in the Practice of Psychiatry. Washington, DC, American Psychiatric Press, 1990

Ekblom B: Acts of Violence by Patients in Mental Hospitals. Uppsala, Sweden, Scandinavian University Books, 1970

Evenson RC, Altman H, Sletten IW, et al: Disturbing behavior: a study of incident reports. Psychiatr Q 48:266–275, 1974

Fine MJ, Acker C: Hoping the law will find an answer. Philadelphia Inquirer, September 13, 1989, p 1Aff

Gutheil TG: Prosecuting patients. Hosp Community Psychiatry 36:1320–1321, 1985

Halleck S: The assessment of responsibility in criminal law and psychiatric practice, in Law and Mental Health: International Perspectives, Vol 1. Edited by Weisstub D. New York, Pergamon Press, 1984, pp 193–220

Hoge SK, Gutheil TG: The prosecution of psychiatric patients for assaults on staff: a preliminary empirical study. Hosp Community Psychiatry 38:44–49, 1987

Hoge SK, Appelbaum PS, Greer A: An empirical comparison of the Stone and dangerousness criteria for civil commitment. Am J Psychiatry 146:170–175, 1989

Johansen KH: The impact of patients with chronic character pathology on a hospital inpatient unit. Hosp Community Psychiatry 34:842–846, 1983

Kalogerakis MG: The assaultive psychiatric patient. Psychiatr Q 45:372–381, 1971

Lanza ML: The reactions of nursing staff to physical assault by patients. Hosp Community Psychiatry 34:44–47, 1983

Lidz CW, Mulvey EP, Appelbaum PS, et al: Commitment: the consistency of clinicians and the use of legal standards. Am J Psychiatry 146:176–181, 1989

Lion JR, Pasternak SA: Countertransference reactions to violent patients. Am J Psychiatry 130:207–210, 1973

Lion JR, Snyder W, Merrill GL: Underreporting of assaults on staff in a state hospital. Hosp Community Psychiatry 32:497–498, 1981

Madden DJ, Lion JR, Penna MW: Assaults on psychiatrists by patients. Am J Psychiatry 133:422–425, 1976

Massachusetts General Laws, Chapter 19, Section 10, effective July 1, 1987

McCall and McCall v Department of Health and Rehabilitative Services, 536 So 2d 1098 (1988)

McNiel DE, Binder RL: Predictive validity of judgments of dangerousness in emergency civil commitment. Am J Psychiatry 144:197–200, 1987

Melick ME, Steadman HJ, Cocozza JJ: The medicalization of criminal behavior among mental patients. J Health Soc Behav 20:228–237, 1979

Miller RD, Maier GJ: Factors affecting the decision to prosecute mental patients for criminal behavior. Hosp Community Psychiatry 38:50–55, 1987

Monahan J, Ruggiero M, Friedlander HD: Stone-Roth model of civil commitment and the California dangerousness standard: operational comparison. Arch Gen Psychiatry 39:1267–1271, 1982

Norko MA, Zonana HV, Phillips RTM: Prosecuting assaultive psychiatric patients. J Forensic Sci 37:923–931, 1992

Packer HL: The Limits of the Criminal Sanction. Stanford, CA, Stanford University Press, 1968

Phelan LA, Mills MJ, Ryan JA: Prosecuting psychiatric patients for assaults. Hosp Community Psychiatry 36:581–582, 1985

Rappeport J: Ethics and forensic psychiatry, in Psychiatric Ethics. Edited by Bloch S, Chodoff P. Oxford, England, Oxford University Press, 1981, pp 255–276

Reich W: Psychiatric diagnosis as an ethical problem, in Psychiatric Ethics. Edited by Bloch S, Chodoff P. Oxford, England, Oxford University Press, 1981, pp 61–88

Schwarz CJ, Greenfield GP: Charging a patient with assault of a nurse on a psychiatric unit. Canadian Psychiatric Association Journal 23:197–200, 1978

State v Cummins, 168 NJ Super 429, 433 A2d 67 (1979)

Steadman HJ, Cocozza JJ, Melick ME: Explaining the increased arrest rate among mental patients: the changing clientele of state hospitals. Am J Psychiatry 135:816–820, 1978

Stein LI, Diamond RJ: The chronic mentally ill and the criminal justice system: when to call the police. Hosp Community Psychiatry 36:271–274, 1985

Tarasoff v Regents of the University of California, 17 Cal 3d 425, 551 P2d 334 (1976)

Tardiff K, Sweillam A: Assaultive behavior among chronic inpatients. Am J Psychiatry 139:212–215, 1982

Turkington D: Litigaphobia: practitioners' exaggerated fear of lawsuits cripples them and does patients a disservice. APA Monitor 17: 1, 8, 1986

United States Sentencing Commission: Sentencing Guidelines and Policy Statements (Chapter 4A1.1). Washington, DC, United States Sentencing Commission, 1992

Whitman RM, Armao BB, Dent OB: Assault on the therapist. Am J Psychiatry 133:426–429, 1976

Index

Page numbers printed in **boldface** *type refer to tables or figures.*